*Get Through*
# MRCOG Part 2: MCQs

To Angela

# Get Through
# MRCOG Part 2: MCQs

**Paul Ayuk** BSc (Hons) MB BS (Hons) PhD MRCOG
Obstetrician and Gynaecologist
John Radcliffe Hospital
Oxford, UK

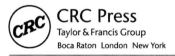

CRC Press
Taylor & Francis Group
Boca Raton  London  New York

CRC Press is an imprint of the
Taylor & Francis Group, an **informa** business

# Contents

# Preface

This book has been written by an obstetrician and gynaecologist who has developed and run an on-line MRCOG training course (www.busyspr.com) for over 5 years. During this time, the course has been used by over 8000 trainees worldwide and their comments, suggestions and constructive criticisms has played a major role in improving the quality of the mateiral used in this book.

The text is organised in 13 chapters covering the entire MRCOG II syllabus plus two mock exams. Every set of questions is followed by answers and brief but detailed explanation notes. Where possible, the notes extend beyond the specific issues assessed in the question, increasing their value as a revision tool.

# 1. Bleeding in pregnancy: Questions

**1.1**   In early pregnancy:

A The yolk sac is the first structure to be identified and disappears by 10 weeks' gestation.

B About 70% of twin pregnancies identified at <10 weeks' gestation result in an ongoing singleton pregnancy.

C The doubling time for HCG is ~72 h.

D Falling HCG concentrations indicate a non-viable pregnancy.

**1.2**   With respect to molar pregnancy:

A Complete moles have a 69XXY karyotype.

B Maternal serum AFP levels are undetectable in complete moles.

C Medical evacuation using prostaglandins and oxytocin is the recommended treatment.

D During surgical evacuation, oxytocin infusion should be commenced before the uterus is empty.

**1.3**   With respect to molar pregnancy:

A Women should be advised not to conceive until HCG levels have been normal for 12 months.

B Use of the combined oral contraceptive pill after HCG levels have returned to normal is associated with increased need for chemotherapy.

C There is a recognized association with ovarian theca-leutein cysts.

D Use of IUDs is contraindicated until after HCG levels have returned to normal.

**1.4**   The following are associated with an increased risk of malignant change in a woman with a molar pregnancy:

A Maternal age over 39 years.

B A woman with blood group A with a partner with blood group O.

C Partial hydatidiform moles.

D Smoking.

1.5    Complete hydatidiform moles:

A Secrete leutenizing hormone.
B Have maternally derived chromosomes.
C Usually have avascular trophoblastic villi.
D May be complicated by hypothyroidism.

1.6    With respect to molar pregnancies:

A Women presenting with persistent vaginal bleeding following evacuation of a complete molar pregnancy should undergo a further uterine evacuation.
B Women with placental site trophoblastic tumour do not need to be registered with a surveillance centre.
C Women should be advised not to become pregnant until HCG levels have reverted to normal for 6 months.
D Mifepristone is recommended for termination of a partial molar pregnancy at 14 weeks' gestation.

1.7    With respect to molar pregnancies:

A Termination of pregnancy should be recommended if a twin pregnancy is diagnosed with one complete molar pregnancy.
B In a twin pregnancy with one molar pregnancy, the chances of a viable fetus are ~10%.
C Ultrasound is a highly sensitive tool in the diagnosis of partial molar pregnancy.
D The presence of cystic spaces in the placenta with a viable fetus is suggestive of a partial molar pregnancy.

1.8    In a woman with choriocarcinoma:

A A rise in the level of urinary HCG after initial clinical response is diagnostic of recurrence.
B There is usually a recent history of first trimester miscarriage.
C With optimal treatment, the 5-year survival rate is <70%.
D Successful chemotherapy is followed by a return of fertility in most young women.

**1.9** With respect to gestational trophoblastic disease:

A Chorioadenoma destruens is typically associated with theca-lutein ovarian cysts.

B HCG levels are invalidated by administration of the oral contraceptive pill.

C 3% of women with complete molar pregnancy develop choriocarcinoma.

D Choriocarcinoma responds to treatment with folic acid antagonists.

**1.10** A 20-year-old, Rhesus-negative and unsensitized woman is found to have a 10 weeks' size missed miscarriage:

A Anti-D immunoglobulin should be administered if surgical evacuation is performed.

B Anti-D immunoglobulin is unnecessary after medical evacuation.

C Screening for *Chlamydia* infection is recommended prior to evacuation.

D Histological examination of products of conception is recommended.

**1.11** The following are recommended investigations in a woman who is otherwise fit and well with three successive first trimester miscarriages:

A Pelvic ultrasound scan.

B Laparoscopy.

C Fasting blood glucose and thyroid function tests.

D Hysteroscopy to exclude uterine anomalies.

**1.12** The following are recognized features of septic miscarriage:

A Hypertension.

B Disseminated intravascular coagulation.

C Acute renal failure.

D Jaundice.

**1.13** The following are associated with an increased risk of first trimester miscarriage:

A PCOS.

B Treated hypothyroidism.

C Well controlled insulin dependent diabetes.

D Balanced translocation in the father.

**1.14** In a woman with a threatened miscarriage at 8 weeks' gestation:

A Vaginal examination should be avoided until after an ultrasound scan.

B Bed-rest is effective treatment.

C Progesterone supplementation has been shown to be effective treatment.

D Anti-D immunoglobulin is recommended in Rhesus-negative unsensitized women.

**1.15** In a woman with three previous second trimester miscarriages:

A Hysteroscopy should be performed to diagnose cervical incompetence.

B A cervical suture should be inserted 10 weeks into her next pregnancy.

C Transvaginal ultrasound scan may be used to diagnose cervical incompetence.

D Randomized trials have shown a definite benefit for cervical cerclage.

**1.16** In a woman with three previous second trimester miscarriages:

A Randomized trials have shown a definite benefit for prophylactic antibiotics.

B Randomized trials have shown that the combination of aspirin and heparin is superior to aspirin alone in improving pregnancy outcome.

C Antiphospholipid antibodies may be positive.

D If a septate uterus is identified, uterine surgery has been shown to improve pregnancy outcome.

**1.17** With respect to cervical incompetence and preterm labour:

A The normal cervical length is 38–42 mm on transvaginal scanning.

B There is an increased risk of preterm delivery associated with a cervical length <38 mm.

C Cervical cerclage has been shown in randomized trials to be associated with a reduction in perinatal mortality.

D Cervical cerclage has been shown to be associated with a increased risk of maternal infection.

**1.18** In the diagnosis of antiphospholipid antibody syndrome, the following are considered as adverse pregnancy outcomes:

    A Two consecutive miscarriages before 10 weeks' gestation.
    B One morphologically normal fetal death after 10 weeks' gestation.
    C One delivery before 34 weeks' gestation.
    D One neonatal death of a term baby.

**1.19** Regarding the diagnosis of ectopic pregnancy:

    A Diagnostic laparoscopy has a false-negative rate of about 4%.
    B Viable intrauterine pregnancies are detectable by transvaginal ultrasound when serum beta-HCG levels are 1000 IU/L.
    C Single serum progesterone measurements are useful in the diagnosis of ectopic pregnancy.
    D Use of colour Doppler can differentiate an incomplete miscarriage from an ectopic pregnancy.

**1.20** Regarding the diagnosis of ectopic pregnancy:

    A Ectopic pregnancy accounts for 1% of all direct maternal deaths.
    B The incidence of ectopic pregnancy in the UK is 0.2%.
    C Mortality from ectopic pregnancy has remained unchanged over the last 20 years.
    D Ectopic pregnancies with a serum beta-HCG of <1000 mIU/L can be managed expectantly.

**1.21** The following are associated with an increased risk of ectopic pregnancy:

    A Ovulation induction using clomephene citrate.
    B Ovulation induction using gonadotrophins.
    C Use of the progesterone-only pill.
    D Smoking.

**1.22** Ectopic pregnancy:

    A Is associated with uterine enlargement.
    B May co-exist with an intrauterine pregnancy.
    C When located in the uterine cornua is associated with a lower risk of haemorrhage.
    D Is located in the ovary in 5% of cases.

**1.23** A 30-year-old woman is found to have an ectopic pregnancy on transvaginal ultrasound scanning:

A Salpingotomy is associated with a significantly greater subsequent intrauterine pregnancy rate compared to salpingectomy.

B Salpingotomy is associated with a greater rate of recurrent ectopic pregnancy compared to salpingectomy.

C During salpingectomy, as small a segment of the fallopian tube as possible should be removed.

D Laparoscopic procedures are more cost-effective compared to laparotomy.

**1.24** Regarding the use of methotrexate in the management of ectopic pregnancy:

A An un-ruptured ectopic pregnancy of <3.5cm diameter can be treated successfully with methotrexate.

B An ectopic pregnancy with fetal cardiac activity is a contra-indication to methotrexate treatment.

C The success rate of single dose methotrexate treatment is about 90%.

D An increase in abdominal pain is a frequent complaint following methotrexate administration.

**1.25** Regarding the use of methotrexate in the management of ectopic pregnancy:

A The intrauterine pregnancy rate following treatment is 30%.

B 20% of subsequent pregnancies are ectopic.

C Recurrent ectopic pregnancy rates are similar to those following laparoscopic salpingostomy.

D Tubal patency tests will be positive in 30% of women following treatment.

**1.26** Regarding the use of methotrexate in the management of ectopic pregnancy:

A Normal trophoblast cells are more sensitive to methotrexate than malignant trophoblast cells.

B Serum beta-HCG levels may increase between days 1 and 4 following methotrexate treatment.

C A rise in serum beta-HCG levels 48 h after methotrexate administration is an indication for surgical treatment.

D Increased abdominal pain following methotrexate administration is an indication for surgical treatment.

1.27   A diagnosis of pregnancy of unknown location:

   A  Can be made at HCG levels >3000 IU/L.
   B  Should not be made if more than 6 weeks have elapsed after the LMP.
   C  Cannot be made if HCG levels are rising.
   D  Can be managed expectantly if the woman is asymptomatic.

1.28   In the management of a pregnancy of unknown location:

   A  Women should initially be followed up every week.
   B  Active intervention should be recommended if HCG levels rise above the discriminatory zone.
   C  Serial HCG levels should be measured until HCG is undetectable.
   D  Up to 75% of women will require active intervention if expectant management is undertaken.

1.29   During expectant management of an ectopic pregnancy:

   A  Serial HCG measurements should be undertaken twice weekly initially.
   B  Transvaginal ultrasound scan should be performed every week initially.
   C  HCG levels should be monitored until they fall below 20 IU/L.
   D  Ideally, HCG levels should rise by <50% in the first 7 days.

1.30   The following are recognized complications of early medical termination of pregnancy with prostaglandins:

   A  Diarrhoea.
   B  Pyrexia.
   C  Bronchospasm.
   D  Hyponatraemia.

1.31   Mifepristone:

   A  Is a 19-keto-steroid and a progesterone antagonist.
   B  Blocks uterine oestrogen receptors.
   C  Can cause severe vaginal bleeding.
   D  May interfere with glucocorticoid function.

**1.32**   Mifepristone:

A  Can be used for medical termination of pregnancy up to 12 weeks' gestation.
B  Can be used with diclofenac as analgesia.
C  Can safely be used in renal failure.
D  Is contraindicated in smokers over the age of 35 years.

**1.33**   Placenta previa:

A  Is associated with an increased risk of fetal congenital anomaly.
B  Is associated with an increased risk of placenta acreta.
C  Is typically associated with vaginal bleeding in the second trimester.
D  Is associated with an increased risk of neonatal hypovolaemic shock.

**1.34**   With regards to placenta previa:

A  Vaginal delivery is recommended if the lower edge of an anterior placenta is 3 cm from the internal os on transvaginal scanning.
B  Caesarean section is indicated if the lower edge of the placenta is within 2 cm of the internal os.
C  Transabdominal scanning is superior to transvaginal scanning in the diagnosis of anterior placenta previa.
D  The risk of placenta acreta is significantly reduced.

**1.35**   With respect to placenta previa:

A  Outpatient management is just as effective as inpatient management in women with grade II placenta previa and no bleeding.
B  If a woman does not wish to have blood transfusion, 2 units of blood may be collected during the antenatal period for autologous transfusion if needed.
C  Neonatal anaemia and hypovolaemia are recognized complications of caesarean section.
D  Antepartum blood loss is fetal in origin.

**1.36**   The following are associated with an increased risk of placenta previa:

A  Previous uterine infection.
B  Teenage pregnancy.
C  Previous caesarean section.
D  Pregnancy associated with IUCD.

1.37    The following are risk factors for placental abruption:

   A  Polyhydramnios.
   B  Oligohydramnios.
   C  Pre-eclampsia.
   D  External cephalic version.

1.38    A 34-year-old woman presents at 34 weeks' gestation with vaginal bleeding and abdominal pain. Her pulse is 100/min and blood pressure 130/70:

   A  An emergency caesarean section should be performed if fetal heart rate decelerations are present.
   B  Maternal blood pressure is a good indicator of blood loss.
   C  Renal failure is a possible complication.
   D  Thrombocytosis is a recognized complication.

1.39    A 30-year-old woman is admitted at 30 weeks' gestation with severe constant abdominal pain. She looks pale with BP 110/70, pulse 100/min. Fetal heart beat is absent. Hb 11 g/dl, platelet count 25 000/ml:

   A  Epidural anaesthesia is contraindicated.
   B  The most likely diagnosis is disseminated sepsis.
   C  Depletion of Factor VIII is likely.
   D  Fibrin degradation product levels are likely to be low.

1.40    A 30-year-old woman is admitted at 30 weeks' gestation with severe constant abdominal pain. She looks pale with BP 110/70, pulse 100/min. Fetal heart beat is absent. Hb 11 g/dl, platelet count 25 000/ml:

   A  Blood transfusion is unlikely to be necessary as her Hb concentration is normal.
   B  Central venous pressure monitoring is indicated.
   C  There is an increased risk of post-partum haemorrhage.
   D  Thromboprophylaxis with heparin is contraindicated post-partum.

# Answers

## 1.1 Answers

**A** **True** – The yolk sac is the first structure that can be accurately identified in the gestation sac; it is visualized at 5–6 weeks from LMP and disappears at about 10 weeks. Max. diameter is 5 mm at ~7 weeks.

**B** **True** – 71% of viable twin pregnancies diagnosed by ultrasound before 10 weeks result in an ongoing singleton pregnancy (vanishing twin).

**C** **False** – An HCG doubling time of ≤2 days in early pregnancy is consistent with an intrauterine pregnancy.

**D** **True** – Falling HCG levels before 10–12 weeks' gestation indicate a non-viable pregnancy.

## 1.2 Answers

**A** **False** – Complete moles have a 46,XX karyotype.

**B** **True** – No fetal parts in complete moles; AFP not produced.

**C** **False.**

**D** **False** – Uterotonic agents should be avoided before the uterus is empty as they may increase the risk of embolization of molar tissue.

## 1.3 Answers

**A** **False** – Women should be advised not to fall pregnant until HCG levels have returned to normal.

**B** **False** – Use of COCP after HCG levels have normalized is not associated with increased requirement for chemotherapy.

**C** **True** – High HCG levels result in ovarian theca-leutein cysts.

**D** **True** – IUDs are contraindicated until HCG levels have returned to normal.

## 1.4 Answers

**A** **True** – A nine-fold increase in risk of malignant change in women >40 years compared to 20–24 age group.

**B** **True** – Highest risk in woman with blood group A and partner with blood group O; lowest risk in woman with blood group A and partner with blood group A.

**C** **False** – There is malignant potential with complete mole; 7–16% require chemotherapy compared to 0.5% after partial mole.

**D** **False.**

Note:
- Lowest risk of malignant change is associated with vacuum aspiration as the initial method of evacuation.
- Post-evacuation COCP use before HCG levels have returned to normal is associated with increased need for chemotherapy.

## 1.5    Answers

**A** **False** – Secrete large quantities of HCG.
**B** **False** – Complete moles have a 46,XX karyotype – caused by a single sperm fertilizing an anucleate oocyte, then duplicating its genetic material.
**C** **True** – Characterized by hydropic avascular villi with a snow-storm appearance on ultrasound scan.
**D** **False** – The alpha subunit of HCG is identical to the alpha subunit of TSH and high levels of HCG may cause symptomatic *hyper*thyroidism.

## 1.6    Answers

**A** **False** – If persistent vaginal bleeding develops after evacuation of a molar pregnancy, advice should be sought from the nearest screening centre before further surgical intervention is undertaken.
**B** **False** – Women with molar pregnancies should be registered with one of the three national screening centres. Criteria for registration include: complete or partial mole, twin pregnancy with complete or partial mole, choriocarcinoma, placental site trophoblastic tumour and microscopic change suggestive of molar pregnancy.
**C** **True** – Women should be advised not to conceive until the HCG level has been normal for 6 months. COCP and HRT are safe to use after HCG levels have reverted to normal.
**D** **False** – Use of mifepristone should be avoided.

Note:
- Medical evacuation may be used in partial molar pregnancies if the size of fetal parts precludes the use of suction evacuation.

## 1.7    Answers

**A** **False** – In twin pregnancy with one viable fetus and the other molar, allow pregnancy to proceed if the woman wishes after appropriate counseling. There is an increased risk of pre-eclampsia and VTE.
**B** **False** – Chances of a viable fetus ~40%.
**C** **False** – Ultrasound diagnosis of partial molar pregnancy is difficult – presence of cystic spaces in the placenta and a transverse anteroposterior diameter of the gestation sac of >1.5 are suggestive.
**D** **True.**

Note:
- Majority of complete molar pregnancies diagnosed as delayed (missed) miscarriages or anembryonic pregnancies. However, typical snowstorm ultrasound appearance may be present.

## 1.8    Answers

**A  False** – It could be a new pregnancy.

**B  False** – 50% of patients will have had a preceding molar pregnancy; 25% of cases follow a spontaneous or induced abortion; and 25% of cases follow a normal or an ectopic pregnancy.

**C  False** – The overall 5-year survival with optimal treatment is 95%.

**D  True** – Approximately 90% of patients who want to become pregnant following chemotherapy have succeeded and there is no evidence of increase in fetal abnormalities.

## 1.9    Answers

**A  True.**

**B  False.**

**C  True** – About 2–3% of hydatidiform moles are complicated by the development of choriocarcinoma.

**D  True.**

Note:
- COCP may increase the risk of requiring chemotherapy if given before HCG levels return to normal.
- Sensitive to chemotherapy with methotrexate but combination chemotherapy is now used.

## 1.10   Answers

**A  True** – Anti-D immunoglobulin should be administered if an intervention is undertaken to evacuate the uterus.

**B  False.**

**C  True** – Screening for genital tract infection with *Chlamydia* is recommended in women below the age of 25 years or those at high risk prior to uterine instrumentation.

**D  True** – Products of conception should be sent for histological examination to exclude molar tissue.

## 1.11   Answers

**A  True.**

**B  False.**

**C  False.**

**D  False.**

Note: Investigation of woman with recurrent miscarriage:

- Karyotype of couple – refer to clinical geneticist if positive result.
- Karyotype of products of conception if next pregnancy fails.
- Pelvic ultrasound scan – ovarian morphology/uterine anomalies.
- Screening for antiphospholipid antibodies on two occasions at least 6 weeks apart – third test if discordant results; treat with low dose aspirin + heparin.
- Screening for inherited thrombophilias.

**1.12 Answers**

**A** False.
**B** True.
**C** True.
**D** True.

Note: Complications of septic miscarriage:

* Endometritis progressing to pelvic cellulitis/abscess and septicaemia.
* Endotoxic shock – features include hypotension, tachycardia, tachypnoea, hypothermia (<35°C) or pyrexia, hypoxaemia, oliguria and positive blood cultures.
* DIC leading to jaundice.
* Crepitus may occur following infection with gas-forming organisms – this usually complicates illegal abortions.

**1.13 Answers**

**A** **True** – Ultrasound features of polycystic ovaries are more prevalent in women with recurrent miscarriage (50%) compared to general population (22%).
**B** **False.**
**C** **False** – Well controlled diabetes mellitus and thyroid disease are not associated with recurrent miscarriage. Incidence of subclinical diabetes mellitus is not higher in recurrent miscarriage. Poorly controlled diabetes mellitus is associated with increased risk of miscarriage.
**D** **True** – 3–5% of couples presenting with recurrent miscarriage carry a chromosomal anomaly, most commonly a balanced translocation. The incidence of balanced translocation in general population is ~0.4%. The female is twice as likely as the male to be a carrier of translocation.

Note:

* Pre-pregnancy suppression of LH in women with LH hypersecretion does not improve outcome.

**1.14 Answers**

**A** **False** – Vaginal examination should be undertaken and there is no evidence that this adversely affects outcome.
**B** **False** – Bed-rest does not improve pregnancy outcome and may be harmful.
**C** **False** – Progesterone supplementation does not improve pregnancy outcome.
**D** **False** – Anti-D immunoglobulin is not recommended and should only be considered if bleeding is heavy and associated with pain.

## 1.15 Answers

**A** **False** – Hysteroscopy is not useful in the diagnosis of cervical incompetence as it cannot be undertaken during pregnancy.

**B** **False.**

**C** **True** – The diagnosis of cervical incompetence is based on clinical obstetric history aided by physical examination and transvaginal ultrasound.

**D** **False** – Randomized trials have shown that cervical cerclage does not improve pregnancy outcome in women in whom the diagnosis of cervical incompetence is uncertain or suggested by transvaginal scanning.

## 1.16 Answers

**A** **False** – Neither prophylactic antibiotics nor cervical cerclage have been shown to improve pregnancy outcome in women with recurrent second trimester loss.

**B** **False** – Aspirin on its own does not improve pregnancy outcome in women with recurrent second trimester pregnancy loss.

**C** **True** – Antiphospholipid antibody syndrome is a recognized cause of recurrent second trimester pregnancy loss.

**D** **False** – Congenital uterine anomalies are not associated with recurrent pregnancy loss and surgical correction is not recommended.

## 1.17 Answers

**A** **True.**

**B** **False** – Cervical length <25 mm is associated with a 50% risk of preterm delivery.

**C** **False** – Cervical cerclage does not improve pregnancy outcome, even in women with shortened cervices on transvaginal scanning.

**D** **True** – Cervical cerclage is associated with an increased risk of puerperal pyrexia and medical intervention, including the use of tocolytics, induction of labour and caesarean section.

## 1.18 Answers

**A** **False** – Three or more miscarriages before 10 weeks.

**B** **True.**

**C** **False** – One or more deliveries before 34 weeks due to severe pre-eclampsia, eclampsia or IUGR.

**D** **False.**

## 1.19 Answers

**A** **True** – Diagnostic laparoscopy has a false-positive rate of 5% and a false-negative rate of 3–4%.

**B** **False** – There is some debate on the level of HCG at which a viable intrauterine gestation sac should be detectable on transvaginal ultrasound scan but most would accept a level of >1500 IU/L.

**C** **False** – Single serum progesterone measurements do not satisfactorily distinguish ectopic from intrauterine pregnancies.

**D** **True.**

## 1.20 Answers

**A** **False** – Ectopic pregnancy accounts for ~10% of all direct maternal deaths.

**B** **False** – Incidence of ectopic pregnancy in the UK is 11.1 per 1000 pregnancies.

**C** **False** – Mortality has decreased four-fold in the last 20 years.

**D** **True** – Expectant management is appropriate if serum HCG levels are below the discriminatory zone (level at which it is assumed that a viable intrauterine pregnancy would be visualized on transvaginal scan: 1000–2000 IU/L).

## 1.21 Answers

**A** **True.**

**B** **True.**

**C** **True** – Affects tubal motility. Risk in women taking mini-pill higher than for COCP but lower than for sexually active women not taking contraception.

**D** **True.**

Note: Risk factors for ectopic pregnancy:

- Previous ectopic pregnancy.
- Tubal surgery/reversal of sterilization.
- Previous PID.
- Use of progesterone-only pill.
- Use of ovulation-inducing agents/IVF.
- Pregnancy with IUCD in situ.
- Smoking.

## 1.22 Answers

**A** **True.**

**B** **True** – Heterotopic pregnancies are rare but incidence is increased with IVF.

**C** **False.**

**D** **False** – 0.5% of cases are ovarian. 0.1% of ectopic pregnancies are intra-abdominal; 2% are corneal and carry a higher risk of haemorrhage. Of tubal pregnancy, 55% ampulla, 17% fimbrial end, 25% isthmus.

## 1.23 Answers

**A** **False** – With both tubes present, there does not appear to be a difference in subsequent intrauterine pregnancy rate (46% vs 44%).

**B** **True** – Recurrent ectopic pregnancy rate appears to be higher after salpingotomy although data are conflicting.

**C** **False** – As much of the tube as possible should be removed during salpingectomy to prevent recurrent ectopic pregnancy.

**D** **True** – Laparoscopy is associated with: lower blood loss, lower analgesic requirement, shorter hospital stay, quicker post-op recovery, lower cost, no significant difference in subsequent intrauterine pregnancy rates, a trend towards a lower repeat ectopic pregnancy rate, and lower risk of adhesion formation.

Note:

- Risk of persistent trophoblastic tissue is higher after salpingotomy than after salpingectomy: monitor HCG levels; risk of tubal bleeding in the immediate post-op period.
- In a haemodynamically stable woman, laparoscopy is preferable to laparotomy.

## 1.24 Answers

**A** **True.**

**B** **True** – The presence of fetal cardiac activity is a contraindication to medical treatment.

**C** **True** – Success rates of 85–94% following single dose methotrexate treatment.

**D** **True** – An increase in abdominal pain is reported by 59% of women following methotrexate administration.

Note: Criteria for medical treatment:

- Ectopic mass <3.5 cm.
- No fetal cardiac activity.
- Initial HCG <3000 IU/L.

## 1.25 Answers

**A** **False** – Among women trying to become pregnant after medical management of ectopic pregnancy, intrauterine pregnancy rate = 54% and recurrent ectopic rates = 8–10%, which are comparable to those following laparoscopic salpingostomy.

**B** **False.**

**C** **True.**

**D** **False** – Ipsilateral tubal patency rates following treatment are ~80%.

## 1.26 Answers

**A** False.

**B** True – Serum beta-HCG should be measured on days 4 and 7.
A further dose of methotrexate should be considered if HCG levels fall by
<15% between days 4 and 7.

**C** False – A transient increase in beta-HCG may occur in up to 86% of
women between days 1 and 4 of treatment.

**D** False – An increase in abdominal pain is reported by 59% of women
following methotrexate.

## 1.27 Answers

**A** False – Serum HCG levels are below the discriminatory zone (level at
which it is assumed that a viable intrauterine pregnancy would be visualized
on transvaginal scan: 1000–2000 IU/L).

**B** False.

**C** False.

**D** True – Women with minimal/no symptoms can be managed expectantly
with 48–72 h follow-up and active management if symptomatic, HCG levels
rise above discriminatory zone or levels plateau.

Note:

• If no pregnancy is detectable on scan, the pregnancy is of unknown location.

## 1.28 Answers

**A** False.

**B** True – Active management if HCG levels rise about the discriminatory
zone or levels plateau.

**C** False – Monitor serum HCG until below 20 IU/L.

**D** False – Intervention may be required in 23–29% of cases.

## 1.29 Answers

**A** True – Perform twice weekly serum HCG levels and weekly transvaginal
scans to ensure levels falling rapidly and size of ectopic mass decreasing.
Thereafter, weekly HCG and scans until HCG <20 IU/L.

**B** True.

**C** True.

**D** False.

Note:

• Criteria for expectant management: asymptomatic and haemodynamically stable;
HCG low and falling (<1000 IU/L); <50–100 ml of blood in pouch of Douglas;
gestation sac <2–5 cm with no FH on scan.

• Low and rapidly falling HCG levels indicate high likelihood of successful expectant
management.

• Provide clear written information on the importance of compliance with follow-up
and easy access to the hospital.

• Rupture may still occur under these circumstances.

### 1.30  Answers

A **True.**
B **True.**
C **True.**
D **False.**

Note: Side effects of prostaglandins:
- Diarrhoea, nausea and vomiting, abdominal cramps.
- Bronchospasm, chest pain and palpitations (not misoprostol) – mifepristone should not be used with gemeprost in smokers over the age of 35 years.
- Pyrexia/chills, flushing.
- Severe hypotension, coronary artery spasm and MI reported.

### 1.31  Answers

A **False** – Derivative of norethindrone (19-norsteroid) – similar chemical structure to progesterone/glucocorticoids; a progesterone/glucocorticoid antagonist.
B **False.**
C **True.**
D **True.**

Note:
- Inhibits negative feedback of cortisol on ACTH secretion resulting in a significant increase in ACTH and cortisol after a single 100 mg dose.
- Side effects: vaginal bleeding, malaise, headache, nausea and vomiting, rash.

### 1.32  Answers

A **False** – Licensed for use in early medical termination of pregnancy up to 63 days from LMP with administration of prostaglandins (oral/vaginal) 36–48 h after mifepristone.
B **False** – Avoid aspirin/NSAIDs for at least 8–12 days after mifepristone.
C **False** – Hepatic/renal failure is a contraindication.
D **True** – Contraindicated in smokers over the age of 35 years (avoid smoking/alcohol 2 days before and on the day of prostaglandin administration).

Note:
- Contraindications to mifepristone: suspected ectopic pregnancy; chronic adrenal insufficiency; long-term corticosteroid therapy; haemorrhagic disorders; anticoagulant therapy, smokers over the age of 35, hepatic/renal impairment.

### 1.33  Answers

A **True** – Incidence of serious congenital malformations doubles in fetuses with placenta previa – mainly cardiovascular, respiratory and gastrointestinal.
B **True** – Placenta acreta occurs in up to 15% of women with placenta previa.
C **False** – Bleeding typically occurs in the third trimester.
D **True** – Fetal hypovolaemia may occur from bleeding during delivery or ruptured vasa previa.

## 1.34 Answers

**A** **True** – Placenta encroaching within 2 cm of the internal os is a contraindication to vaginal delivery.

**B** **True.**

**C** **False** – Transabdominal scanning is associated with a high number of false-positive diagnoses of placenta previa, especially with a posterior placenta. Transvaginal scanning is safe and superior to transabdominal scanning.

**D** **False** – Risk of placenta acreta is increased in women with placenta previa, especially in women with a previous caesarean section.

## 1.35 Answers

**A** **False** – Inpatient management is recommended for women with major placenta previa in the third trimester.

**B** **False** – There is no evidence to support the use of autologous blood transfusion in women with placenta previa – patients may require up to 18 units of blood.

**C** **True** – Neonatal anaemia and hypovolaemia occur secondary to fetal blood loss during delivery or ruptured vasa previa.

**D** **False** – APH from placenta previa is maternal blood but fetal blood loss can occur as in C.

## 1.36 Answers

**A** **True.**

**B** **False** – Risk increases with increasing maternal age.

**C** **True** – Single C/S, risk increased by 0.65%; four or more C/S, risk increased by 10%.

**D** **False.**

Note:

• Risk factors for placenta previa: increased maternal age, increased parity; previous C/S, smoking; previous placenta previa (recurrence risk 4–8% after one previa), previous uterine infection.

## 1.37 Answers

**A** **True** – Sudden uterine decompression after membrane rupture – polyhydramnios, multiple pregnancy.

**B** **False.**

**C** **True** – Association with hypertension is controversial but risk is increased in pre-eclampsia.

**D** **True** – Uterine/abdominal trauma is a risk factor, including ECV.

Note:

• Risk factors for placental abruption: uterine/abdominal trauma, previous abruption – recurrence risk 8–17%; older maternal age (due to increasing parity rather than maternal age per se); smoking, sudden uterine decompression after membrane rupture, pre-eclampsia.

### 1.38 Answers

A **True** – Delivery is indicated if there is evidence of maternal or fetal compromise.

B **False** – Maternal BP is a poor indicator of blood loss and hypotension is a late sign.

C **True.**

D **False.**

Note:
- The most important diagnosis is placental abruption. This diagnosis should be made if pain is constant.
- Fetal complications include: prematurity, hypoxic injury, fetal death.
- Maternal complications include: shock, DIC (with thrombocytopaenia), renal failure, complications of operative delivery, PPH.

### 1.39 Answers

A **True** – In the presence of a coagulopathy or thrombocytopenia, regional anaesthesia is contraindicated.

B **False** – The most likely diagnosis is a concealed abruption.

C **True** – Low platelet count suggests DIC – clotting factors, including Factor VIII, will be low and FDP concentration will be elevated.

D **False** – See C.

### 1.40 Answers

A **False** – Current Hb concentration is likely to be an overestimate as blood loss is recent. Blood transfusion is likely to be required.

B **True.**

C **True** – PPH is a recognized complication of placental abruption, especially in the presence of DIC.

D **False** – Associated with increased risk of VTE and thromboprophylaxis should be commenced once the risk of haemorrhage is assessed to have diminished.

# 2. Medical disorders and pregnancy: Questions

2.1　In pregnant epileptics on phenytoin:

A　Increased protein binding occurs.
B　Reduction in plasma levels is mainly due to increased liver metabolism.
C　There is an increased risk of neural tube defects.
D　Maternal vitamin K is recommended from 36 weeks' gestation.

2.2　In pregnant epileptics on phenytoin:

A　Neonatal vitamin K is recommended.
B　Breastfeeding should be discouraged.
C　There is a recognized fetal syndrome.
D　Pre-pregnancy folic acid (0.4 mg) is recommended.

2.3　Phenytoin:

A　Is best administered by i.m. injection.
B　Has a short half-life in vivo.
C　Is readily absorbed from the gut.
D　Is metabolized by the liver.

2.4　Phenytoin:

A　Causes hypoglycaemia in diabetic women.
B　Serum levels are increased by acute alcohol intake.
C　Serum levels are decreased by chronic alcohol intake.
D　Is highly protein bound.

2.5　With respect to thyroid function and thyroid disease in pregnancy:

A　Only 10% of hyperthyroidism is due to Graves' disease.
B　Graves' disease usually worsens in the third trimester.
C　Symptoms of Graves' disease may worsen in the puerperium.
D　Biopsy of a solitary thyroid nodule should be deferred until after delivery.

2.6    Hyperthyroidism is associated with:

A  Increased risk of preterm delivery.
B  Increased risk of stillbirth.
C  Increased risk of fetal macrosomia.
D  Fetal craniosynostosis.

2.7    In a woman with well-controlled Graves' disease:

A  There is no increased risk of neonatal thyroid disease.
B  Neonatal hypothyroidism may occur.
C  Neonatal hyperthyroidism may occur.
D  There is an increased risk of recurrent miscarriage.

2.8    With respect to thyrotoxicosis in pregnancy:

A  Breastfeeding is contraindicated in women taking propylthiouracil.
B  Neonatal thyrotoxicosis is clinically apparent within 24 hours of delivery.
C  Antithyroid drugs should be replaced by beta-blockers from 36 weeks' gestation.
D  Drug treatment can be reliably monitored by the sole use of serial serum total thyroxine concentration.

2.9    With respect to thyrotoxicosis in pregnancy:

A  Thyroid enlargement indicates inadequate treatment.
B  Mild thyrotoxicosis cannot be distinguished clinically from normal pregnancy.
C  Subtotal thyroidectomy is acceptable treatment in the second trimester.
D  Neonatal hyperthyroidism does not occur if the mother has been euthyroid.

2.10   With respect to thyrotoxicosis in pregnancy:

A  Neonatal goitre is a recognized complication of over-treatment.
B  Administration of a blocking dose of carbimazole plus thyroxine replacement is appropriate treatment.
C  Radio-iodine thyroid scans are contraindicated in pregnancy.
D  Radio-iodine thyroid scans are contraindicated in breastfeeding women.

**2.11**   With respect to thyrotoxicosis in pregnancy:

A   Fetal thyrotoxicosis in a euthyroid woman should be treated by maternal administration of antithyroid drugs plus thyroxine replacement.

B   Pregnancy should be avoided for at least 4 months after radio-iodine treatment.

C   Neonatal thyrotoxicosis carries a 1% mortality rate if untreated.

D   In a woman with newly diagnosed thyrotoxicosis, beta-blockers should be continued for the rest of the pregnancy.

**2.12**   Graves' disease in pregnancy:

A   Becomes progressively more active as pregnancy advances.

B   Frequently gets worse in the puerperium.

C   May cause neonatal hyperthyroidism in 1–2%.

D   Thyroid-stimulating antibodies are IgM.

**2.13**   Hypothyroidism in pregnancy:

A   Can safely be treated with oral carbimazole.

B   May be associated with antithyroid antibodies.

C   May lead to neonatal hypothyroidism.

D   Is commoner in Caucasian than African populations.

**2.14**   In women with systemic lupus erythematosus:

A   Spontaneous miscarriage is more common.

B   Premature delivery is more common.

C   IUGR is more common.

D   Neonatal SLE may occur.

**2.15**   A 30-year-old woman is known to have the antiphospholipid antibody syndrome:

A   Her risk of deep venous thrombosis is increased.

B   Her risk of stroke is increased.

C   Her risk of miscarriage is reduced by treatment with prednisolone.

D   The combined oral contraceptive pill is absolutely contraindicated.

**2.16** The following are known to cause acute renal failure:

A Malaria.
B Sickle cell trait.
C Septicaemia.
D Concealed antepartum haemorrhage.

**2.17** Renal glomerular function may be accurately assessed by the following measurements:

A Plasma urate.
B Plasma bicarbonate.
C Plasma urea.
D Creatinine clearance.

**2.18** In a pregnant woman with chronic renal disease:

A The presence of squamous epithelial cells on microscopic examination of urine is characteristic.
B Urine protein excretion is increased.
C Creatinine clearance is increased.
D Pregnancy significantly affects the natural history of renal disease.

**2.19** In a pregnant woman with a functioning renal transplant:

A The risk of acute rejection is increased during pregnancy.
B Pregnancy adversely affects long-term renal function.
C Azathioprine is associated with congenital anomalies.
D Vaginal delivery is recommended.

**2.20** In a pregnant woman with a functioning renal transplant:

A Pelvic osteodystrophy is a recognized complication of renal failure and dialysis.
B There is an increased risk of pre-eclampsia.
C ACE inhibitors are contraindicated.
D If taking oral prednisolone, hydrocortisone should be prescribed during labour.

**2.21** The following may cause acute pre-renal renal failure in pregnancy:

A Antepartum haemorrhage.
B Post-partum haemorrhage.
C Incompatible blood transfusion.
D Hyperemesis gravidarum.

**2.22** Renal acute cortical necrosis:

    A Is more common in the pregnant compared to the non-pregnant.

    B Is most frequently associated with placental abruption.

    C Characteristically follows post-partum haemorrhage.

    D Is a more common cause of acute renal failure than acute tubular necrosis.

**2.23** In pregnancy complicated by asthma:

    A There is an increased risk of congenital malformations.

    B High-dose oral corticosteroids are contraindicated.

    C There is an increased perinatal mortality rate.

    D Premature labour is less common.

**2.24** Amniotic fluid embolism:

    A Is always a postmortem diagnosis.

    B Requires the finding of fetal cells in the maternal lungs.

    C Can occur antepartum.

    D Causes rapid hypofibrinogenaemia.

**2.25** With respect to glucose metabolism in pregnancy:

    A Fasting blood glucose concentrations are higher than in the non-pregnant.

    B Plasma insulin concentrations are higher than in the non-pregnant.

    C Insulin resistance increases rapidly after delivery of the placenta.

    D Maternal hyperglycaemia is associated with fetal acidosis.

**2.26** The following screening tests have a high sensitivity (>90%) in the detection of gestational diabetes:

    A Detection of glycosuria.

    B Random glucose measurement.

    C Fasting glucose measurement.

    D Measurement of glycosylated haemoglobin.

**2.27** In gestational diabetes:

    A Maternal islet cell damage is a causal factor.

    B Congenital anomalies are more common.

    C Maternal insulin requirements increase after delivery.

    D Neonatal hyperglycaemia is common.

**2.28** In pregnancy complicated by maternal insulin-dependent diabetes mellitus:

A There is an increased risk of neural tube defects.
B There is an increased incidence of Down syndrome.
C Insulin requirements fall after delivery.
D Insulin crosses the placenta and causes fetal hyperinsulinaemia.

**2.29** In pregnancy complicated by maternal insulin-dependent diabetes mellitus:

A There is decreased perinatal mortality.
B There is an increased incidence of shoulder dystocia.
C Oral hypoglycaemics should be considered if glycaemic control is difficult.
D There is an increased risk of neonatal hyperglycaemia and hypocalcaemia.

**2.30** In pregnancy complicated by maternal insulin-dependent diabetes mellitus:

A Folic acid 0.4 mg should be commenced pre-pregnancy.
B The risk of intrauterine death of the fetus is highest in the last 4 weeks of pregnancy.
C Biophysical profile score accurately predicts intrauterine death.
D There is an increased risk of congenital cardiac anomalies.

**2.31** In pregnancy complicated by maternal insulin-dependent diabetes mellitus:

A Neonatal respiratory distress syndrome is less common.
B There is an increased risk of neonatal jaundice.
C There is an increased risk of neonatal hypocalcaemia.
D There is an increased risk of neonatal hypermagnesaemia.

**2.32** In gestational diabetes:

A Neonatal jaundice is more common.
B There is an increased risk of shoulder dystocia.
C Corticosteroids have been shown to improve fetal lung maturity.
D Induction of labour is recommended at 37 weeks' gestation.

**2.33** The following conditions have increased incidence in pregnancy associated with poorly controlled IDDM:

A Acute pyelonephritis.
B Fetal oesophageal atresia.
C Preterm labour.
D Sacral agenesis.

**2.34** Gestational diabetes is associated with:

A An increased risk of diabetes mellitus in the woman in later life.
B A need for insulin treatment in the majority of cases.
C An increased risk of fetal malformations even when adequately treated.
D Neonatal hypercalcaemia.

**2.35** In patients with gestational diabetes mellitus:

A There is a positive family history (first-degree relation) in about 25% of cases.
B Less than 2% will develop impaired glucose tolerance within 5 years.

**2.36** With respect to maternal complications of diabetes mellitus in pregnancy:

A Improved glycaemic control may result in worsening of retinopathy.
B Nephropathy typically presents with a derangement of serum creatinine and electrolytes.
C Nausea and vomiting may be due to autonomic neuropathy.
D ACE inhibitors are recognized therapy in the treatment of hypertension.

**2.37** Anaemia in pregnancy:

A The MCV is the most sensitive indicator of iron deficiency anaemia.
B Serum ferritin is increased.
C Red cell folate is a more sensitive indicator of folate deficiency.
D A normal MCV excludes folate deficiency.

**2.38** Anaemia in pregnancy:

A Is associated with nulliparity.
B Vitamin $B_{12}$ deficiency is associated with a megaloblastic picture.
C Increased lobulation of the nuclei of neutrophils occurs with folate deficiency.
D MCV is increased in thalassaemia.

**2.39** Sickle cell disease in pregnancy is associated with:

A IUGR.
B Neonatal sickle cell crisis.
C Increased risk of pre-eclampsia.
D Fat embolism.

**2.40** In a pregnant woman with sickle cell disease, the following are consistent with acute chest syndrome:

A Pyrexia.
B Increased white cell count.
C Pleuritic chest pain.
D Tachypnoea.

**2.41** Features of sickle cell–haemoglobin C disease in pregnancy include:

A A characteristic association with anaemia.
B Splenomegaly.
C Bone infarction.
D Fat embolism.

**2.42** Features of sickle cell–haemoglobin C disease in pregnancy include:

A Increased risk of thromboembolism.
B An increased risk of puerperal sepsis.
C No risk of acute chest syndrome.
D Increased risk of haemorrhagic stroke.

**2.43** Recognized features of sickle cell disease complicating pregnancy include:

A Increased risk of iron deficiency.
B Fat embolism.
C Increased risk of venous thromboembolism.
D Splenic sequestration.

**2.44** Recognized features of sickle cell disease complicating pregnancy include:

A Increased risk of pneumonia.
B Four-fold increase in perinatal mortality in the UK.
C A need for vitamin C supplementation.
D Increased risk of folate deficiency.

**2.45** Thalassaemia major is:

A A microcytic hypochromic variety of anaemia.
B Caused by heterozygous inheritance of thalassaemia genes.
C Associated with secondary amenorrhoea.
D Associated with fetal hydrops in a fetus with beta-thalassaemia.

**2.46** Cholestasis of pregnancy:

A Characteristically presents in the second trimester.
B Typically presents with itching over the scalp and abdomen.
C Is associated with an increased risk of preterm labour.
D Is associated with fetal distress in labour.

**2.47** Cholestasis of pregnancy:

A Is associated with meconium-stained liquor.
B Is a diagnosis of exclusion.
C Should be managed by induction of labour at 40 weeks' gestation.
D Is associated with unconjugated hyperbilirubinaemia.

**2.48** Cholestasis of pregnancy:

A Serum bile acid concentrations are usually within the normal range.
B Steatorrhoea, dark urine, malaise and epigastric discomfort may occur.
C Acute fatty liver of pregnancy is a known complication.
D Ursodeoxycholic acid is licensed for use in pregnancy.

**2.49** Acute fatty liver of pregnancy:

A Affects 1:2000 pregnancies.
B Is more common if the woman is carrying a female fetus.
C Is associated with hypoglycaemia.
D Typically presents with collapse and epigastric pain.

**2.50** Acute fatty liver of pregnancy:

A Presents before 30 weeks' gestation in the majority of cases.
B The liver ultrasound scan may be normal.
C Should be managed by prompt delivery of the fetus.
D May be complicated by hepatic encephalopathy.

**2.51** Liver disease in pregnancy:

A Jaundice is most commonly caused by viral infections.
B HELLP syndrome does not occur in the absence of hypertension and proteinuria.
C Cholestasis of pregnancy is effectively treated with ursodeoxycholic acid.
D Gilbert's syndrome presents with jaundice.

**2.52** Recognized causes of vomiting in late pregnancy include:

A Ulcerative colitis.
B Red degeneration of uterine fibroid.
C Acute fatty liver of pregnancy.
D Multiple pregnancy.

**2.53** Hyperemesis gravidarum:

A Is associated with urinary tract infection.
B Is uncommon before 12 weeks' gestation.
C May be associated with jaundice.
D May be associated with abnormal liver enzymes.

**2.54** Hyperemesis gravidarum:

A Is characteristically associated with hypokalaemia.
B Is a diagnosis of exclusion.
C In severe cases may be complicated by Wernicke's encephalopathy.
D Is typically associated with hypertension.

**2.55** With respect to hyperemesis gravidarum:

A The severity is directly related to serum HCG concentration.
B Wernicke's encephalopathy is a recognized complication.
C There is an association with transient hypothyroidism in ~5% of women.
D Metabolic alkalosis is a recognized complication.

**2.56** Pulmonary embolism:

    A Is the second commonest direct cause of maternal mortality in the UK.

    B Is typically preceded by symptomatic DVT.

    C Should only be treated with anticoagulants following definitive diagnosis using a V/Q scan.

    D Should be treated with heparin only during the antenatal period.

**2.57** Pulmonary embolism:

    A Is associated with maternal sinus bradycardia.

    B Causes hypoxia and hypercapnia on maternal blood gas analysis.

    C Is associated with a respiratory alkalosis.

    D Is associated with signs of right-sided heart strain on ECG.

**2.58** A 30-year-old woman with a previous DVT is planning a pregnancy:

    A Low molecular weight heparin should be started at 6 weeks' gestation if she has no other risk factors.

    B If she has an inherited thrombophilia, low molecular weight heparin should be started pre-pregnancy.

    C If she is heterozygous for Factor V Leiden mutation, low molecular weight heparin should be started as soon as she is pregnant.

    D If she has antithrombin deficiency, antenatal thromboprophylaxis is not currently recommended.

**2.59** A 30-year-old woman with a previous DVT is planning a pregnancy:

    A If the previous DVT was related to the OCP, antenatal thromboprophylaxis is unnecessary.

    B Her risk per day of recurrent VTE is maximal in the puerperium.

    C Antenatal thromboprophylaxis is recommended if she had an axillary vein thrombosis.

    D She should be advised that if she requires a caesarean section, general anaesthesia would be recommended.

**2.60** With respect to VTE in pregnancy:

A The majority of fatal antenatal pulmonary embolisms occur in the first trimester.

B The majority of post-partum deaths from VTE follow vaginal delivery.

C The pro-thrombotic changes associated with pregnancy reach their peak during the third trimester.

D Most VTE occurs post-partum.

**2.61** A 35-year-old woman has just had a normal vaginal delivery:

A Thromboprophylaxis with LMW heparin is recommended for 3–5 days if she has a previous DVT but no thrombophilia.

B If she is heterozygous for Factor V Leiden but has no previous VTE, LMW heparin is not recommended.

C If she has a BMI of 40 kg/m², LMW heparin should be considered for 3–5 days.

D LMW heparin may safely be administered before the epidural catheter is removed.

**2.62** In a 30-year-old primigravida with mitral valve prolapse without regurgitation:

A Routine induction of labour at 40 weeks is recommended.

B The second stage should be electively shortened.

C Ergometrine is contraindicated in the third stage.

D Antibiotic cover to prevent bacterial endocarditis is not recommended following a normal vaginal delivery.

**2.63** With regards to heart murmurs in pregnancy:

A Diastolic murmurs occur in over 50% of pregnant women.

B The majority of diastolic murmurs are innocent flow murmurs.

C In the absence of symptoms, echocardiography is normal in over 90% of cases of systolic murmurs.

D The left sternal border is most frequently the area of maximum intensity.

**2.64** Regarding peripartum cardiomyopathy:

A Cerebral embolization is a major cause of morbidity.

B Cardiac transplantation is inappropriate.

C The mortality rate within the first year is >80%.

D Anticoagulation is required.

**2.65** Regarding peripartum cardiomyopathy:

A The condition is more common in nulliparous women.
B It typically occurs in women with rheumatic heart disease.
C It is associated with an increased risk of venous thromboembolism.
D It is an obstructive cardiomyopathy.

**2.66** The following are characteristic skin manifestations of normal pregnancy:

A Palmar erythema.
B Pemphigoid.
C Vitiligo.
D Spider naevi.

**2.67** Pemphigus:

A Can be aggravated by pregnancy.
B Is associated with an increased fetal death rate.
C Is associated with neonatal skin lesions.
D Methotrexate and azathioprine are recognized therapies.

**2.68** Ehlers–Danlos syndrome in pregnancy is associated with:

A An increased risk of post-partum haemorrhage.
B An increased risk of gestational diabetes.
C An increased risk of wound dehiscence.
D An increased risk of maternal mortality.

**2.69** With regards to psoriasis in pregnancy:

A The disease is usually unaffected by pregnancy.
B Generalized pustular psoriasis carries a poor fetal prognosis.
C Corticosteroids are contraindicated in generalized pustular psoriasis.
D Arthritis is a recognized manifestation.

**2.70** A pregnant woman presents with an itchy rash at 30 weeks' gestation:

A Onset and prominence of the rash in abdominal striae is consistent with polymorphic eruption of pregnancy.

B Involvement of the umbilicus is consistent with pemphigoid gestationis.

C The presence of bullae is consistent with polymorphic eruption of pregnancy.

D Polymorphic eruption of pregnancy usually spares the scalp, face, palms and mucous membranes.

**2.71** A pregnant woman presents with an itchy rash at 30 weeks' gestation:

A Pemphigoid gestationis is associated with other autoimmune diseases.

B Polymorphic eruption of pregnancy is characterized by the deposition of complement in cutaneous basement membrane.

C Polymorphic eruption of pregnancy is associated with poor perinatal outcome.

D Oral antihistamines may safely be administered.

**2.72** Pemphigoid (herpes) gestationis:

A Is caused by infection with the herpes simplex virus.

B Is an autoimmune disorder.

C Characteristically gets worse within 24–48 hours after delivery.

D May present in the post-partum period.

**2.73** Pituitary microadenomas:

A Are <10 cm in diameter.

B Usually do not produce symptoms in pregnancy.

C The majority are prolactin-secreting adenomas.

D Decrease in size during pregnancy.

**2.74** Regarding the pituitary–adrenal axis and steroid production in pregnancy:

A ACTH levels are higher in pregnancy compared to the non-pregnant state.

B Cortisol binding globulin levels are elevated in pregnancy.

C Serum free cortisol levels are unchanged in pregnancy.

D The placenta produces ACTH and corticotrophin-releasing hormone.

**2.75** The following drugs may exacerbate skeletal muscle weakness in a woman with myasthenia gravis:

A Magnesium sulphate.
B Ritodrine.
C Prostaglandin gel.
D Aminoglycosides.

**2.76** In a pregnant woman with myasthenia gravis:

A Double vision may be a presenting symptom.
B Symptoms usually improve postnatally.
C The first stage of labour is prolonged.
D Epidural anaesthesia is contraindicated.

**2.77** In a pregnant woman with myasthenia gravis:

A Respiratory compromise may occur during labour.
B Acute exacerbations should be treated with atropine.
C Neonatal respiratory compromise and feeding difficulties may occur.
D Polyhydramnios is a recognized complication.

**2.78** In a pregnant woman with rheumatoid arthritis:

A The disease is exacerbated by pregnancy.
B Relapse is likely to occur after delivery.
C There is a marked increase in the risk of IUGR.
D The risk of pre-eclampsia is increased.

**2.79** Phaeochromocytoma complicating pregnancy:

A Is characteristically associated with paroxysmal hypertension.
B Is associated with increased urinary excretion of 5-hydroxyindoleacetic acid.
C Is usually sited in the adrenal cortex.
D Causes obstetric collapse.

**2.80** Peptic ulcer disease:

A Is more common during pregnancy.
B In pregnancy, is associated with *Helicobacter pylori* in ~30% of cases.
C Is more commonly diagnosed during pregnancy than in the non-pregnant.
D In pregnancy should be treated by triple therapy.

**2.81** With respect to inflammatory bowel disease during pregnancy:

    A Metronidazole is the recommended treatment for acute exacerbation of Crohn's disease in the first trimester.

    B Ulcerative colitis developing for the first time during pregnancy is likely to be severe.

    C Active Crohn's disease is commonly associated with megaloblastic anaemia.

    D Treatment with sulfasalazine is contraindicated.

**2.82** With respect to inflammatory bowel disease during pregnancy:

    A Ulcerative colitis remains quiescent in over 50% of women.

    B Azathioprine therapy is associated with significant embryopathy.

    C If relapse occurs during pregnancy, it is most likely to occur in the third trimester.

    D In a woman with quiescent ulcerative colitis at conception, the risk of relapse during pregnancy is about 30%.

**2.83** Coeliac disease in pregnancy:

    A Is typically associated with folic acid malabsorption.

    B Should be treated with a phenylalanine-free diet.

    C The prothrombin time should be checked in the third trimester.

    D If untreated, is associated with recurrent miscarriage.

**2.84** Coeliac disease in pregnancy:

    A If untreated, is associated with an increased risk of neural tube defects.

    B Is caused by sensitivity to gluten.

    C Is associated with an increased risk of neonatal hypercalcaemia.

    D Is associated with vitamin K malabsorption.

**2.85** There is a recognized association between disseminated intravascular coagulation and:

    A Placenta previa.

    B Multiple pregnancy.

    C Iron-deficiency anaemia.

    D Prolonged bed rest.

2.86 Features of disseminated intravascular coagulation include:

A Activation of factor VII.
B An association with SLE.
C The appearance of free plasmin in the circulation.
D Reversal of the process by transfusion of stored whole blood.

2.87 With respect to immunosupressive drugs in pregnancy:

A Prednisolone does not cross the placenta.
B Azathioprine is a pro-drug.
C The fetal liver converts azathioprine to 6-mecarptopurine.
D Tacrolimus does not cross the placenta.

2.88 The following drugs are contraindicated in pregnancy:

A Augmentin.
B Insulin.
C Warfarin.
D Heparin.

2.89 The following drugs are absolutely contraindicated in pregnancy:

A Lithium.
B Betamethasone.
C Prednisolone.
D Thyroxine.

2.90 The following drugs are contraindicated in breastfeeding:

A Nalidixic acid.
B Rifampicin.
C Senna.
D Lithium carbonate.

2.91 The use of low-dose aspirin in pregnancy:

A Aspirin inhibits platelet thromboxane synthesis.
B Aspirin secreted in milk may be harmful to the babies of breastfeeding mothers.
C Randomized trials have shown a benefit in women with a previous history of pre-eclampsia.
D Is an alternative to heparin in women with a history of DVT.

2.92 The following are characteristic of the fetal hydantoin syndrome:

A Cleft lip/palate.
B Hypertelorism.
C Atrioventricular septal defect.
D Broad nasal bridge.

2.93 The following are characteristic features of the fetal warfarin syndrome:

A Nasal hypoplasia.
B Microcephaly.
C Hydrocephalus.
D Cardiac anomalies.

2.94 The following drugs are teratogenic:

A Warfarin.
B Phenytoin.
C Heparin.
D Azathioprine.

2.95 The following conditions are exacerbated in pregnancy:

A Sickle cell disease.
B Irritable bowel syndrome.
C Eisenmenger's syndrome.
D Multiple sclerosis.

2.96 Immune thrombocytopenia:

A Can be effectively treated with intravenous gamma-globulin.
B Is best treated with splenectomy.
C Carries a significant risk of fetal haemorrhage.
D Does not usually respond to steroids.

2.97 The following are recognized complications of massive blood transfusion:

A Polycythaemia.
B Thrombocytosis.
C Iron overload.
D Hypokalaemia.

# Answers

### 2.1 Answers

**A False** – Decreased protein binding occurs during pregnancy resulting in increased free drug concentrations.

**B True** – Phenytoin is hydroxylated in the liver by an enzyme system which is saturable at high plasma levels – increased drug metabolism and excretion in pregnancy.

**C True** – Increased risk of neural tube defects with use of antiepileptics.

**D True** – Vitamin K recommended from 36 weeks' gestation. Hepatic enzyme-inducing drugs increase the risk of vitamin K deficiency and haemorrhagic disease in the neonate.

### 2.2 Answers

**A True.**

**B False** – Breastfeeding should not be discouraged. Most antiepileptic drugs are present in breast milk only in very low concentrations.

**C True** – Causes fetal hydantoin syndrome – cleft lip/palate, hypertelorism, broad nasal bridge, hypoplasia of distal phalanges and nails, IUGR, learning disability.

**D False** – Pre-conception folic acid 5 mg.

### 2.3 Answers

**A False** – Readily absorbed from the gut, therefore administered orally.

**B False** – The plasma half-life after oral administration averages 22 h.

**C True.**

**D True** – Most of the drug is metabolized by the liver and excreted in the bile as inactive metabolites.

### 2.4 Answers

**A False** – Has been reported to cause hyperglycaemia in diabetics.

**B True** – Acute alcohol intake increases phenytoin concentrations.

**C True** – Chronic alcohol use results in induction of hepatic enzymes and a reduction in serum concentrations.

**D True.**

### 2.5 Answers

**A False** – 90% of cases are due to Graves' disease – secondary to autoimmune thyroid stimulating antibodies (IgG antibodies), which cross the placenta.

**B False** – Symptoms may improve in third trimester.

**C True** – Risk of post-partum exacerbation.

**D False** – Because of the possibility of malignancy, a solitary thyroid nodule should be investigated during pregnancy.

**2.6** **Answers**

**A** True.
**B** True.
**C** False.
**D** True.

Note:
• Fetal and neonatal risks of hyperthyroidism: neonatal thyrotoxicosis, low birth weight, increased risk of stillbirth and preterm delivery, craniosynostosis, exophthalmos, heart failure.

**2.7** **Answers**

**A** **False** – Neonatal hyperthyroidism may occur in euthyroid women with Graves' disease.
**B** **True** – Antithyroid drugs cross the placenta and may cause neonatal hypothyroidism.
**C** **True** – Thyroid-stimulating antibodies cross the placenta and can cause hyperthyroidism (1–10% risk).
**D** **False** – Treated thyroid disease is not associated with miscarriage.

**2.8** **Answers**

**A** **False** – Breastfeeding is not contraindicated; the concentration of PTU in breast milk is very low.
**B** **False** – Neonatal symptoms may not present for up to a week after delivery.
**C** **False** – Antithyroid drugs should be used throughout pregnancy. Discontinue beta-blockers after symptomatic improvement.
**D** **False** – T4 total and T3 increase in pregnancy. Monitoring requires free T3/T4 and TSH.

**2.9** **Answers**

**A** **False** – Thyroid enlargement occurs in normal pregnancy and may also be a sign of malignancy.
**B** **True** – Many symptoms are similar to symptoms of normal pregnancy, making clinical diagnosis unreliable.
**C** **False** – Surgery should only be undertaken in women with suspected malignancy, pressure symptoms or allergy to antithyroid agents.
**D** **False** – Neonatal hyperthyroidism can occur in women with adequately treated Graves' disease.

**2.10** **Answers**

**A** **True** – Antithyroid drugs cross the placenta and over-treatment may result in fetal hypothyroidism and goitre.

**B** **False** – There is *no* place for 'block and replace' regimens.

**C** **True.**

**D** **False** – While diagnostic radio-iodine scans are contraindicated in pregnancy, they may be undertaken if breastfeeding and breastfeeding is stopped for 24 hours. Avoid pregnancy for at least 4 months after radio-iodine treatment.

**2.11** **Answers**

**A** **True** – If the mother is euthyroid, treat with antithyroid drugs and maternal thyroxine replacement.

**B** **True.**

**C** **False** – Neonatal hyperthyroidism carries a mortality rate up to 50%.

**D** **False** – Discontinue beta-blockers once symptoms improve.

**2.12** **Answers**

**A** **False** – Like other autoimmune disorders, symptoms improve with advancing pregnancy with a tendency to relapse after delivery.

**B** **True.**

**C** **True** – Neonatal hyperthyroidism in 1–10% of cases which may present up to 7 days after birth.

**D** **False** – Thyroid-stimulating antibodies are IgG and cross the placenta.

**2.13** **Answers**

**A** **False.**

**B** **True** – Antithyroid antibodies may cause neonatal hypothyroidism.

**C** **True.**

**D** **True** – Incidence is 9 (Caucasian) and 3 (Black) per 1000 pregnant women.

Note:
- Hypothyroidism is more common than hyperthyroidism in pregnancy.
- Commonest cause is autoimmune (idiopathic), including Hashimoto's thyroiditis.
- Associated with thyroid microsomal antibodies.

**2.14** **Answers**

**A** **True.**

**B** **True** – Increased risk of preterm delivery although the risk of preterm labour is not increased.

**C** **True.**

**D** **True** – Neonatal lupus erythrematosus occurs in ~1:20 000 neonates and is associated with heart block, skin and haematological abnormalities.

Note:
- Fetal/neonatal risks with SLE: miscarriage, fetal death in uteron, IUGR, preterm delivery, neonatal lupus erythematosus.

## 2.15 Answers

**A True** – Women with antiphospholipid syndrome are at increased risk of arterial and venous thrombosis.

**B True.**

**C False** – Corticosteroids do not improve pregnancy outcome in women with antiphospholipid syndrome.

**D True.**

Note:

- Primary antiphospholipid syndrome is the association between antiphospholipid antibodies and adverse pregnancy outcome or vascular thrombosis.
- Adverse pregnancy outcomes include three or more consecutive miscarriages before 10 weeks, one or more morphologically normal fetal deaths after 10 weeks or one or more preterm deliveries before 34 weeks due to pre-eclampsia or IUGR.
- A combination of aspirin and heparin significantly improves live birth rates in women with recurrent miscarriage and antiphospholipid syndrome.
- Treatment with aspirin alone does not seem to improve live birth rates but there remains some controversy.

## 2.16 Answers

**A True.**

**B False.**

**C True.**

**D True** – APH/PPH.

Note: Causes of acute renal failure are:

- Haemorrhage.
- Sepsis.
- Volume depletion – pre-eclampsia, hyperemesis.
- Haemolysis – HELLP, malaria, pre-eclampsia, acute fatty liver of pregnancy, haemolytic uraemic syndrome, incompatible blood transfusion.
- Drugs – NSAIDs, antibiotics such as aminoglycosides.
- Ureteric damage or obstruction.
- Adrenocortical failure, usually due to inadequate steroid cover.

## 2.17 Answers

**A False** – Renal glomerular function is assessed by creatinine clearance.

**B False.**

**C False** – Serum urea and electrolyte abnormalities are late indicators of renal impairement.

**D True.**

## 2.18 Answers

A **False** – Urine microscopy is characterized by the presence of red blood cells and red cell casts.

B **True** – 24-hour urine protein excretion is increased.

C **False** – Creatinine clearance is decreased.

D **False** – In the majority of women, pregnancy does not influence the natural history of chronic renal disease. However, there is controversy about women with IgA nephropathy, reflux nephropathy and membranoproliferative glomerulonephritis.

## 2.19 Answers

A **False** – The risk of acute rejection is not increased by pregnancy. However, it is recommended that pregnancy should be delayed for at least 2 years after transplant.

B **False** – Pregnancy does not adversely affect long-term renal function.

C **False** – Azathioprine and cyclosporine are not teratogenic. The risk of low birth weight may be increased.

D **True** – The transplanted kidney does not obstruct labour.

## 2.20 Answers

A **True.**

B **True** – ~30% increased risk.

C **True.**

D **True** – All women receiving long-term oral corticosteroids should have steroid cover during labour and delivery.

Note:
- Renal transplantation is associated with increased incidence of caesarean section due to pelvic osteodystrophy secondary to previous renal failure, dialysis or prolonged steroid therapy. The transplanted kidney does not obstruct vaginal delivery.

## 2.21 Answers

A **True** – APH, PPH and miscarriage can cause acute pre-renal failure in pregnancy.

B **True.**

C **True** – Incompatible blood transfusion causes renal failure secondary to haemolysis, haemoglobinuria, hypotension and DIC.

D **True.**

Note:
- Causes of acute pre-renal failure: haemorrhage, hyperemesis gravidarum, septic shock, adrenocortical failure, usually secondary to inadequate steroid cover in women on long-term corticosteroid therapy, and incompatible blood transfusion.

## 2.22 Answers

**A** **True** – Renal acute cortical necrosis is a rare complication and almost always associated with pregnancy, especially in association with placental abruption in older multiparous women.

**B** **True.**

**C** **False.**

**D** **False** – Renal failure from acute tubular necrosis is more common (75% of acute renal failure) and is reversible.

Note:

- Renal acute cortical necrosis is characterized by renal cortical cell death with sparing of the medullary portion of the kidney. If the entire renal cortex is involved, renal failure is irreversible.

## 2.23 Answers

**A** **False** – Asthma is not associated with anomalies.

**B** **False** – Use of inhaled and oral corticosteroids is safe in pregnancy. Steroid cover is required in labour or caesarean section.

**C** **False** – Overall, perinatal mortality/morbidity and risk of preterm delivery are not increased in asthmatics.

**D** **False.**

Note:

- Asthma may improve, worsen or remain unchanged during pregnancy – severe asthma is likely to worsen in late pregnancy.

## 2.24 Answers

**A** **False** – Over 80% mortality.

**B** **False** – Criteria for diagnosis include acute hypotension or cardiac arrest, acute hypoxia, coagulopathy, onset during labour, C/S or within 30 min of delivery and absence of other potential explanations for the above presentation.

**C** **True.**

**D** **True.**

Note:

- Incidence 1:80 000 deliveries.
- Passage of amniotic fluid and debris into the maternal circulation causes an anaphylactic-type reaction.
- Risk factors include increasing maternal age, hypertonic uterine contractions, use of uterotonic agents, induction of labour and uterine trauma.
- If diagnosed before death, management is supportive – give $O_2$, maintain circulation, treat DIC and manage in ITU. Discuss heparin therapy with haematologist.
- Fetal survival is 79% with 39% neurologically intact.

## 2.25 Answers

    **A** **False** – Beta-cell hyperplasia and increased insulin production and secretion occur under the influence of oestrogen and progesterone. As a result, fasting glucose levels are lower in pregnancy compared to non-pregnancy while insulin concentrations are higher.

    **B** **True.**

    **C** **False** – Pregnancy is associated with 'insulin resistance' caused by increasing concentrations of HPL, progesterone and cortisol. Insulin resistance falls rapidly after delivery.

    **D** **True** – Hyperglycaemia and hyperinsulinaemia result in increased fetal aerobic and anaerobic metabolism with hypoxia and lactic acidosis.

## 2.26 Answers

    **A** **False** – Testing for glycosuria has a poor sensitivity in detecting gestational diabetes – only ~40% of women with a 2-h GTT >11 mmol/L have glycosuria in the third trimester.

    **B** **False** – Random blood glucose has a poor sensitivity (~40%) in detecting gestational diabetes.

    **C** **False** – Measurement of fasting glucose on a population basis is difficult and has a low specificity.

    **D** **False** – Measurement of HbA1c also has low sensitivity.

Note:

- Screening for gestational diabetes is controversial. The cost-effectiveness of population screening is principally dependent on the prevalence of gestational diabetes and the acceptability of the screening test.

## 2.27 Answers

    **A** **False** – Gestational diabetes is secondary to insulin resistance and the diabetogenic effects of placental hormones.

    **B** **False** – Gestational diabetes is not associated with congenital anomalies.

    **C** **False** – Insulin resistance falls rapidly after delivery and insulin is not required after delivery.

    **D** **False** – Neonatal hypoglycaemia is a recognized complication.

## 2.28 Answers

    **A** **True** – Congenital anomalies are increased 2–5-fold, especially neural tube defects, cardiac anomalies (transposition of the great vessels), renal anomalies and sacral agenesis (caudal regression syndrome).

    **B** **False** – Risk of aneuploidy is not increased.

    **C** **True** – Insulin requirements increase during pregnancy and fall after delivery.

    **D** **False** – Insulin does not cross the placenta.

## 2.29 Answers

**A** **False** – Maternal IDDM is associated with increased perinatal mortality – congenital anomalies/preterm delivery.

**B** **True** – Macrosomia is associated with an increased risk of shoulder dystocia.

**C** **False** – No role for oral hypoglycaemics in the management of IDDM in pregnancy.

**D** **False** – Increased risk of neonatal hypoglycaemia due to hyperinsulinaemia.

## 2.30 Answers

**A** **False** – Increased risk of neural tube defects; use 5 mg folic acid rather than 0.4 mg.

**B** **True** – Five-fold increased risk of intrauterine death; risk highest in last 4 weeks of pregnancy.

**C** **False** – Fetal hypoxia and acidosis are thought to be initiated by increased aerobic and anaerobic metabolism induced by hyperinsulinaemia and hyperglycaemia with increased production of lactic acid. BPP score does not accurately predict risk.

**D** **True** – 2–5-fold increased risk, especially neural tube defects, cardiac anomalies (transposition of the great vessels), renal anomalies and sacral agenesis (caudal regression syndrome).

## 2.31 Answers

**A** **False** – Increased risk of respiratory distress syndrome, though precise mechanism is unknown.

**B** **True.**

**C** **True** – Caused by fetal beta-cell hyperplasia and neonatal hyperinsulinaemia, and elimination of maternal glucose supply following clamping of the cord.

**D** **False** – Increased risk of *hypo*magnesaemia.

## 2.32 Answers

**A** **True.**

**B** **True.**

**C** **False** – Diabetics were excluded in RCTs on corticosteroids and fetal lung maturity.

**D** **False** – In well-controlled diabetes, delivery should be after 38 weeks' gestation.

Note:
- In gestatational diabetes there is increased risk of: neonatal hypoglycaemia, respiratory distress syndrome, hypocalcaemia and hypomagnesaemia, polycythaemia, neonatal jaundice, fetal macrosomia and shoulder dystocia.

## 2.33 Answers

**A** **True.**
**B** **False** – IDDM is not associated with oesophageal atresia.
**C** **True** – Risk of polyhydramnios is increased with spontaneous preterm labour.
**D** **True.**

Note:
- Poorly controlled IDDM is associated with increased risk of maternal UTI and fetal anomalies, including sacral agenesis and cardiac defects.

## 2.34 Answers

**A** **True** – There is an increased risk of developing diabetes in later life and GTT should be repeated 6–12 weeks post-partum.
**B** **False** – The majority of women can be treated with diet alone.
**C** **False** – No association with an increased risk of fetal anomaly.
**D** **False** – Associated with neonatal *hypo*calcaemia and hypomagnesaemia.

## 2.35 Answers

**A** **True** – A family history of type II diabetes – maternal or sibling but not paternal. Positive family history is present in 25–30% of women.
**B** **False** – 70% life-time risk of type II diabetes (10% general population); 5–10% life-time risk of type I diabetes – women have a slowly progressive form of type I diabetes which is unmasked by pregnancy.

Note:
- There is a recurrence risk of about 66%.

## 2.36 Answers

**A** **True** – Retinopathy may deteriorate in pregnancy in association with improved glycaemic control. Regular ophthalmic assessment with laser treatment as required.
**B** **False** – Nephropathy presents with proteinuria. Serum creatinine and electrolytes usually remain within normal limits.
**C** **True** – Autonomic neuropathy may present with persistent nausea and vomiting (gastropathy).
**D** **False.**

Note:
- Detect and treat hypertension/change medication – discontinue ACE inhibitors (impair fetal renal function), beta-blockers associated with fetal growth restriction.

### 2.37 Answers

**A** **False** – Fall in MCV is the first indication of iron deficiency outside pregnancy but may be normal in the early stages in pregnancy.

**B** **False** – As iron deficiency develops, serum ferritin falls first followed by serum iron. Fall in Hb is a late development.

**C** **True** – Plasma folate shows considerable day-to-day variation. Red cell folate gives a better index of overall body and tissue levels.

**D** **False** – Normal MCV does not exclude folate deficiency – in combination with iron deficiency, MCV can be normal.

### 2.38 Answers

**A** **False** – Iron deficiency is more common in multiparous women.

**B** **True** – Serum $B_{12}$ levels fall in pregnancy and are lower in smokers while $B_{12}$ binding capacity is increased in pregnancy. Deficiency is associated with megaloblastic anaemia as is folate deficiency.

**C** **True** – Hypersegmentation of neutrophil polymorphs is characteristic of folate deficiency but is also observed in pure iron deficiency anaemia.

**D** **False** – MCV is reduced in haemoglobinopathies such as thalassaemia and sickle cell disease.

### 2.39 Answers

**A** **True** – Sickle cell diseases is associated with increased risk of IUGR, spontaneous miscarriage, premature labour, pre-eclampsia (early onset with accelerated course), fetal distress and C/S.

**B** **False.**

**C** **True.**

**D** **True.**

Note:

- Increased perinatal mortality (4–6-fold).
- Two-fold increase in maternal mortality: increased risk of UTI, chest infection, puerperal pyrexia, venous thromboembolism, fat embolism and bone necrosis.
- Folic acid deficiency may lead to megaloblastic anaemia. Iron deficiency is not typical.

### 2.40 Answers

**A** **True.**

**B** **True.**

**C** **True.**

**D** **True.**

Note:

- Features of acute chest syndrome: fever, tachypnoea, pleuritic chest pain, leukocytosis, pulmonary infiltration.

## 2.41 Answers

A **False.**
B **True.**
C **True.**
D **True.**

Note: See 2.42.

## 2.42 Answers

A **True.**
B **True.**
C **False.**
D **False.**

Note:
- HbC disease is a milder variant of HbSS.
- Associated with normal/near-normal Hb levels.
- Risk of massive, sometimes fatal, sickling crisis in pregnancy, especially in the puerparium.
- Sickling may be complicated by bone necrosis, fat embolism, painful crises and acute chest syndrome. Splenic sequestration, renal papillary necrosis and stroke also occur.

## 2.43 Answers

A **False** – Iron deficiency is not typical.
B **True.**
C **True.**
D **True.**

Note: See 2.39.

## 2.44 Answers

A **True.**
B **True** – Increased perinatal mortality (4–6-fold). Two-fold increase in maternal mortality.
C **False.**
D **True** – Folic acid deficiency may lead to megaloblastic anaemia.

Note: See 2.39.

## 2.45 Answers

A **True** – Microcytic hypochromic blood picture.
B **True** – Beta or alpha, autosomal recessive inheritance.
C **True** – Associated with primary and secondary amenorrhoea, growth failure, delayed puberty.
D **False** – Fetal Hb does not have a beta chain and beta-thalassaemia major does not present until a few months after birth.

49

### 2.46 Answers

**A** **False** – Usually presents after 30 weeks with pruritis; worsens as pregnancy progresses and relieved within 48 hours of delivery.
**B** **False** – Palms/soles, limbs and trunk.
**C** **True** – Increased risk of preterm labour, stillbirth, antepartum and intrapartum fetal distress, meconium-stained liquor. 10–20% risk of obstetric haemorrhage (vitamin K mal-absorption).
**D** **True.**

Note:
- Caused by intrahepatic cholestasis.

### 2.47 Answers

**A** **True** – Associated with meconium-stained liquor, IUD, intrapartum fetal distress and preterm delivery.
**B** **False** – Diagnosis based on raised serum bile acids. Conjugated bilirubin and liver enzymes are also raised.
**C** **False** – Induction of labour at 36–38 weeks' gestation.
**D** **False** – Conjugated bilirubin and liver enzymes are raised.

### 2.48 Answers

**A** **False** – Serum bile acid concentrations are markedly raised. Conjugated bilirubin and liver enzymes are also raised.
**B** **True** – Malaise, steatorrhoea, epigastric discomfort, dark urine and anorexia may be present.
**C** **False.**
**D** **False** – Ursodeoxycholic acid reverses biochemical abnormalities but there is no evidence that it alters fetal outcome. Not licensed for use in pregnancy.

Note:
- Cholestasis is the most common pregnancy-induced liver disorder and the second commonest cause of jaundice in pregnancy (after viral hepatitis).

### 2.49 Answers

**A** **False** – Incidence ~1:10 000 pregnancies.
**B** **False** – More common with male fetuses (3x).
**C** **True** – Biochemistry: hypoglycaemia, hyperuricaemia, raised liver enzymes.
**D** **False** – Typically presents in the third trimester with malaise, anorexia, nausea and vomiting, and epigastric pain.

## 2.50 Answers

**A** **False** – see 2.49 D.

**B** **True** – Ultrasound scan shows fatty infiltration of the liver although it may be normal.

**C** **True** – Prompt delivery after correcting coagulopathy and hypoglycaemia.

**D** **True** – Liver failure and encephalopathy are recognized complications.

Note:

- Management of acute fatty liver in pregnancy involves multidisciplinary care involving hepatologist and ITU physician.

## 2.51 Answers

**A** **True** – Worldwide, viral hepatitis is the commonest cause of liver disease in pregnancy.

**B** **False** – HELLP syndrome may occur in women without hypertension or proteinuria. Usually, hypertension and/or proteinuria are not marked.

**C** **False** – Ursodeoxycholic acid acts by altering the bile acid pool and reducing the proportion of hydrophobic and hepatotoxic bile acids. Reduces serum bile acid concentration. Not licensed for use in pregnancy. No evidence that it affects fetal outcome in obstetric cholestasis.

**D** **True** – Gilbert's syndrome presents as mild fluctuating jaundice which may only be apparent when the patient is tired, dehydrated or starved.

Note:

- Gilbert's syndrome is associated with unconjugated hyperbilirubinaemia but liver enzymes are normal.
- Relatively common in Caucasians with prevalence of 1–2%.

## 2.52 Answers

**A** **False.**

**B** **True** – Acute pain, e.g. from red degeneration, adnexal torsion, is associated with vomiting in late pregnancy.

**C** **True** – Acute fatty liver of pregnancy, HELLP syndrome and severe pre-eclampsia are associated with vomiting.

**D** **False.**

Note:

- UTIs are common in pregnancy and their presentation usually includes nausea and vomiting.
- GI disorders including gastroenteritis, viral hepatitis and surgical abdomen should be considered.

## 2.53 Answers

**A** **False** – UTI is a differential diagnosis.

**B** **False** – Hyperemesis is uncommon after 12 weeks.

**C** **True** – Associated with abnormal LFT and jaundice; exclude viral hepatitis.

**D** **True.**

### 2.54 Answers

**A** **True** – Persistent vomiting causes hypokalaemia.

**B** **True** – There is no test that positively confirms the diagnosis which is made after exclusion of UTI, bowel obstruction and endocrine disorders.

**C** **True** – Thiamine deficiency may rarely lead to Wernicke's encephalopathy.

**D** **False** – Dehydration causes postural hypotension.

### 2.55 Answers

**A** **False** – Aetiology not fully understood but related to HCG and TSH levels $\pm$ psychological factors. There is, however, no direct relationship between the severity of the disorder and HCG or TSH levels.

**B** **True** – Wernicke's encephalopathy may occur due to thiamine deficiency – diplopia, ataxia, confusion and abnormal ocular movements.

**C** **False.**

**D** **True** – Associated with metabolic alkalosis – hypochloraemic alkalosis with hypokalaemia and potassium loss in urine.

Note:

• Urine is acidic despite systemic alkalosis – when alkalosis is associated with volume depletion, bicarbonate is not excreted. Excretion of bicarbonate only occurs with restoration of extracellular fluid volume.

### 2.56 Answers

**A** **False** – VTE is the commonest direct cause of maternal mortality in the UK.

**B** **False** – Most women with fatal PE do not have a preceding diagnosis of DVT.

**C** **False** – The puerperium is the most hypercoagulable period. Women with antenatal VTE should be anticoagulated for at least 6 weeks after delivery.

**D** **True** – Warfarin is teratogenic and is associated with risk of fetal haemorrhage. Heparin does not cross the placenta and should be used for antenatal treatment.

### 2.57 Answers

**A** **False.**

**B** **False** – Hypoxia with *hypo*capnia.

**C** **True** – Manifestations of non-fatal PE include: respiratory alkalosis, collapse, pleuritic chest pain, shortness of breath, haemoptysis, tachycardia (sinus on ECG), hypoxia with hypocapnia.

**D** **True** – Signs of right-sided heart strain on ECG, although these may be obscured by pregnancy changes.

**2.58**  **Answers**

- **A** **False** – Low molecular weight heparin for 6 weeks *after* delivery in a woman with previous VTE and no thrombophilia.
- **B** **False** – Use antenatal LMW heparin for at least 6 weeks post-partum in women with an inherited thombophilia.
- **C** **True** – Risk of VTE varies with type of thrombophilia: relative risk of 7 for Factor V Leiden, 2.9–9.5 for prothrombin G20210A, 10–13 for antithrombin, protein C or S deficiency, and 107 for a combination of Factor V Leiden and prothrombin G20210A.
- **D** **False** – Women with more than one VTE, one VTE plus VTE in a first-degree relative or VTE in an unusual site should receive antenatal thromboprophylaxis continued for 6 weeks post-partum.

**2.59**  **Answers**

- **A** **False** – Value of antenatal thromboprophylaxis is controversial. However, if the previous VTE was oestrogen related (pregnancy or OCP) or high BMI, antenatal thromboprophylaxis should be considered.
- **B** **True** – Most VTE occurs antenatally but the risk per day is greatest in the weeks immediately following delivery.
- **C** **True** – See 2.58D.
- **D** **False** – Previous VTE is not a contraindication to regional anaesthesia in labour.

**2.60**  **Answers**

- **A** **True** – 8/13 fatal antenatal PTEs occurred in the first trimester. 10/14 post-partum deaths followed vaginal delivery.
- **B** **True**.
- **C** **False**.
- **D** **False** – See 2.59B.

**2.61**  **Answers**

- **A** **False** – Previous VTE and no thrombophilia: LMW heparin for 6 weeks after delivery.
- **B** **False** – Inherited thrombophilia but no previous VTE: manage according to risk profile.
- **C** **True** – Women without VTE or thrombophilia: assess for risk factors for VTE and consider for LMW heparin for 3–5 days post-partum.
- **D** **True** – Post-partum, heparin should be started as soon as possible if there is no PPH; 4 hours after insertion or removal of epidural catheter. First dose can be given after insertion but before removal.

Note:

- Antenatal and post-partum thromboprophylaxis recommended for women with antithrombin deficiency, those who are homozygous for defects and those with multiple defects. Otherwise post-partum prophylaxis for 6 weeks is recommended.

**2.62   Answers**

**A** False.
**B** False.
**C** False.
**D** True.

Note:

- Common (prevalence 2–4%). Prevalence in women of reproductive age up to 20%.
- Associated with palpitations, syncope, arrhythmias, chest pain and panic attacks.
- Serious complications include severe mitral regurgitation, infective endocarditis, cerebral ischaemia and sudden death.
- In the absence of mitral regurgitation, the risks are minimal. Small risk of supraventricular tachycardia.
- Endocarditis prophylaxis is not recommended for normal delivery.

**2.63   Answers**

**A** **False** – Systolic murmurs are common (prevalence >90%); vast majority are flow murmurs.
**B** **False** – Diastolic mumurs are uncommon and should be considered abnormal as should pansystolic and long and loud systolic murmurs.
**C** **True** – Over 90% of patients have normal cardiac structure and function on echo.
**D** **True.**

**2.64   Answers**

**A** **True** – Venous and arterial thromboembolism: emboli from dilated left ventricle or fibrillating atrium.
**B** **False** – Cardiac transplantation if deterioration continues.
**C** **False** – Mortality rate is 7–50%. 50% of deaths occur within 3 months of delivery.
**D** **True** – Anticoagulate because of risk of arterial and venous thromboembolism.

Note:

- Cause of dilated cardiomyopathy is unknown.
- Prevalence 1:1500 to 1:15 000 live births.
- Aim for vaginal delivery.

**2.65**  **Answers**

> **A** False.
> **B** False.
> **C** True – See 2.64A.
> **D** False.

Note:
- Criteria for diagnosis: cardiac failure in the last month of pregnancy or within 5 months of delivery; no previous cardiac disease; no identifiable cause for cardiac failure; evidence of systolic dysfunction.
- Presentation: dyspnoea with reduced exercise tolerance, cough, dizziness, orthopnoea, palpitations, chest pain. Symptoms may be similar to normal pregnancy symptoms. BP usually normal. JVP raised, arrhythmias, cardiomegaly, hepatomegaly, ascites.

**2.66**  **Answers**

> **A** **True** – Palmar erythema and spider naevi are normal skin changes in pregnancy associated with hyperoestrogenaemia and hyperdynamic circulation.
> **B** **False** – Pemphigoid gestationis is a specific inflammatory dermatoses of pregnancy and is associated with other autoimmune diseases.
> **C** **False** – Vitiligo is an autoimmune disease associated with loss of cutaneous pigmentation.
> **D** **True** – See A.

**2.67**  **Answers**

> **A** True.
> **B** **True** – Possible increased risk of adverse perinatal outcome – monitor fetal growth and wellbeing.
> **C** **True** – 5% of neonates may develop bullous lesions.
> **D** **True** – Treat with topical corticosteroids and oral antihistamines or oral prednisolone in severe cases in pregnancy, although methotrexate and azathioprine are used in non-pregnant.

Note:
- Presents with clusters of vesicles and bullae and is associated with other autoimmune diseases and HLA-B8 and DR3.
- Starts within umbilicus and spreads to involve limbs, palms and soles.
- May improve in later pregnancy but 50–75% experience exacerbation within 24–48 hours of delivery.

**2.68**  **Answers**

> **A** **True** – Types I and IV Ehlers–Danlos syndrome are associated with increased risk of PPH, poor wound healing, wound dehiscence, uterine lacerations and abdominal hernias.
> **B** False.
> **C** True.
> **D** **True** – Maternal mortality up to 25% in type IV.

### 2.69 Answers

**A** **True** – May improve, worsen or remain unchanged during pregnancy.

**B** **True** – Generalized pustular psoriasis presents with sterile pustules, maternal pyrexia and systemic illness which may be complicated by cardiac and renal failure and carries a poor fetal outlook.

**C** **False** – Prompt response to corticosteroids.

**D** **True** – Arthropathy is a recognized feature of psoriasis.

Note:

• Dithranol and coal tar can safely be used in pregnancy.

### 2.70 Answers

**A** **True** – Polymorphic eruption of pregnancy typically begins in abdominal striae as erythematous oedematous papules. Typically spares scalp, face, palms, soles and mucous membranes. Bullae do not occur.

**B** **True** – Pemphigoid gestationis is a specific inflammatory dermatosis of pregnancy. Rare and associated with other autoimmune disorders. Mean gestation at onset is 21 weeks. 20% present post-partum. Lesions first develop in the umbilicus and spread to the trunk and limbs.

**C** **False** – See A.

**D** **True** – See A.

### 2.71 Answers

**A** **True** – Pemphigoid (herpes) gestationis presents with clusters of vesicles and bullae and is associated with other autoimmune diseases and HLA-B8 and DR3.

**B** **False** – Characterized by deposition of complement in cutaneous basement membrane on direct immunofluorescence.

**C** **False** – Polymorphic eruption of pregnancy is not an autoimmune disease and is not associated with adverse fetal outcome.

**D** **True** – Antihistamines can safely be used in pregnancy.

### 2.72 Answers

**A** **False.**

**B** **True.**

**C** **True** – Pemphigoid (herpes) gestationis may improve in later pregnancy but 50–75% experience exacerbation within 24–48 h of delivery.

**D** **True** – Mean gestational age at onset = 21 weeks; 20% present post-partum.

### 2.73 Answers

**A** **False** – <10 mm in diameter.

**B** **True.**

**C** **True** – Majority are prolactin-secreting and are asymptomatic during pregnancy.

**D** **False** – The pituitary and adenomas increase in size during pregnancy.

## 2.74 Answers

**A** **False** – ACTH levels are lower in pregnancy compared to non-pregnant but increase with increasing gestation.

**B** **True** – Serum cortisol levels increase 2–3-fold by term. There is an oestrogen-induced increase in production of cortisol-binding globulin. Free serum cortisol and urinary free cortisol are however also increased in pregnancy.

**C** **False** – See B.

**D** **True** – The placenta produces both ACTH and CRH. The relationship between these placental hormones and maternal adrenal function is unknown.

## 2.75 Answers

**A** **True.**

**B** **False.**

**C** **False.**

**D** **True.**

Note:

- Drugs exacerbating skeletal muscle weakness in myasthenia gravis: magnesium salts, aminoglycosides, propranolol, tetracycline, barbiturates, lithium salts, penicillamine, quinine, procainamide, halothane, polymyxin B.

## 2.76 Answers

**A** **True** – Occular weakness with double vision is a typical presentation. Difficulties with chewing or talking also occur.

**B** **False** – Risk of post-partum exacerbation.

**C** **False** – Smooth muscle not affected, therefore first stage of labour is not altered.

**D** **False** – Patients are particularly sensitive to neuromuscular drugs and anaesthetic review is recommended. Epidural is recommended.

## 2.77 Answers

**A** **True** – Myasthenic crisis requiring ventilation may be precipitated by the stress of labour and delivery, inadvertent change in medication or surgery.

**B** **False** – Atropine is a muscarinic antagonist – nicotinic receptors are affected in myasthenia gravis.

**C** **True** – Transplacental passage of antibodies may cause neonatal myasthenia gravis with poor suckling, feeble cry and respiratory difficulties.

**D** **True** – Swallowing difficulties in the fetus.

### 2.78 Answers

**A** **False** – Characteristically improves during pregnancy with relapse in the puerperium.

**B** **True.**

**C** **False** – No effect on risk of pre-eclampsia, IUGR or preterm delivery.

**D** **False.**

Note:
- Rheumatoid arthritis is an autoimmune disease affecting mainly the small joints and is characterized by exacerbations and remissions.
- Extra-articular manifestations include pleurisy, pericarditis, subcutaneous nodules, pulmonary fibrosis.
- Impact of disease on risk of miscarriage and IUD is controversial.

### 2.79 Answers

**A** **True** – Hypertension including complications like cerebral haemorrhage and cardiac failure. Hypertension may be paroxysmal.

**B** **False** – Increased urinary 5-HIAA occurs in carcinoid tumours.

**C** **False** – Rare tumour of adrenal chromaffin cells or sympathetic nervous tissue. 90% located in adrenal medulla.

**D** **True** – Circulatory collapse after delivery or hypertensive response to anaesthesia.

Note:
- Malignancy occurs in 10% (90% benign) of cases and can only be diagnosed when metastases are present.
- Diagnosis in the antenatal period is associated with ~10% mortality (55% if post-partum diagnosis). Bilateral in 10%.
- Fetal loss rate 15–50%.
- Associated with neurofibromatosis and multiple endocrine neoplasia.
- Presentation: hypertension including complications like cerebral haemorrhage and cardiac failure; postural fall in BP in 50% of cases; headache, abdominal pain, visual symptoms, anxiety, palpitations, chest pain, polyuria (due to glycosuria); circulatory collapse after delivery or hypertensive response to anaesthesia.
- Differential diagnoses: pregnancy-induced hypertension and thyrotoxicosis.
- Elevated urinary excretion of catecholamines and their metabolites, such as vanilly-mandelic acid, is diagnostic. False-positive results may occur in women on methyldopa or labetalol.

### 2.80 Answers

**A** **False** – Decreased frequency of diagnosis of peptic ulcer disease in pregnancy. Incidence of ulcer complications in women with known ulcers also reduced in pregnancy.

**B** **False** – Prevalence of *H. pylori* in peptic ulcer disease is 85–100%.

**C** **False** – Symptoms of peptic ulcer disease tend to reduce during pregnancy. Ulcer symptoms and complications may increase in the puerperium.

**D False** – Therapy for *H. pylori* infection consists of 2 weeks of one or two effective antibiotics, such as amoxicillin, tetracycline (contraindicated in pregnancy), metronidazole or clarithromycin, plus either ranitidine bismuth citrate, bismuth subsalicylate or a proton pump inhibitor. The safety of such therapy in pregnancy has not been established. Medical treatment should be with non-absorbable antacids and H2 antagonists. Concerns about antiandrogenic effects of cimetidine on a male fetus.

Note:
- Peptic ulcer disease in pregnancy is associated with risk of perforation, haemorrhage and obstruction.
- Relapse rate is high because of high prevalence of *H. pylori*.

## 2.81 Answers

**A False.**

**B False** – May first present during pregnancy – course no more severe than in women who develop disease outside pregnancy but diagnosis may be delayed.

**C True** – Crohn's disease especially is associated with increased risk of prematurity. Associated with folate malabsorption and megaloblastic anaemia.

**D False** – Reassure that drug therapy during pregnancy (corticosteroids, sulfasalazine, azathioprine) is safe and continue treatment during pregnancy. Methotrexate, cyclosporine, tacrolimus and mycophenolate-mofetil should be avoided in pregnancy.

Note:
- Steroid enema is not contraindicated in inflammatory bowel disease.

## 2.82 Answers

**A True** – Risk of relapse is not affected by pregnancy. Active disease in early pregnancy is more likely to be associated with relapse in later pregnancy or puerperium.

**B False** – See 2.81D.

**C False** – If relapse occurs, more likely in the first trimester or the puerperium.

**D True** – For ulcerative colitis, 70% of women in remission at conception remain in remission, 20% relapse in first, 7% in second and 1% in third trimester; 3% relapse in puerperium.

Note:
- Active disease at conception is associated with a doubling of the risk of miscarriage.
- In Crohn's disease, 85% of patients in remission remained in remission during pregnancy, 13% relapsed during first trimester, 1% in second and third trimester and ~2% in puerperium.

### 2.83 Answers

**A** True.
**B** False – Treatment by gluten-free diet. See 2.84 B.
**C** True – See 2.84D.
**D** True – See 2.84A.

### 2.84 Answers

**A** True – Untreated or poorly treated coeliac disease is associated with delayed menarche, amenorrhoea, subfertility, recurrent miscarriage, neural tube defects (folate deficiency), anaemia (iron and folate deficiency) and osteomalacia. Fetus at risk of neonatal hypocalcaemia.
**B** True – Gluten enteropathy – sensitivity to dietary gluten (protein component of wheat and other cereals) leads to villous atrophy of the small bowel and malabsorption.
**C** False – Fetus at risk of neonatal *hypo*calcaemia.
**D** True – Vitamin K malabsorption may lead to coagulopathy. Check PT at 36 weeks and administer vitamin K if necessary.

Note:
- Incidence 1:3000.
- Presents with malaise, diarrhoea, weight loss and malabsorption syndromes.
- Endomysial and antigliadin antibodies are useful but small bowel biopsy is required for definitive diagnosis.
- Strict pre-pregnancy control with supplementation of folic acid, iron, and B vitamins.
- Monitor vitamin and iron replacement during pregnancy.

### 2.85 Answers

**A** False.
**B** False.
**C** False.
**D** False.

Note:
- DIC is a thrombohaemorrhagic disorder with production of intravascular fibrin and consumption of clotting factors and platelets.
- Always a secondary disorder associated with: obstetric haemorrhage – APH (typically placental abruption) or PPH, severe pre-eclampsia, sepsis, amniotic fluid embolism, retained dead fetus, acute fatty liver of pregnancy, incompatible or massive blood transfusion, major trauma, molar pregnancy, exacerbations of SLE.

## 2.86 Answers

A **True.**

B **True** – DIC may occur during exacerbations of SLE.

C **True** – Thrombin and plasmin are activated and their balance determines whether a bleeding or thrombotic tendency predominates. Thrombin cleaves fibrinogen to form fibrin monomers and leads to small- and large-vessel thrombosis with ischaemia and organ failure. Plasmin degrades fibrin into measurable degradation products (FDP/D-dimers).

D **False** – Use of fresh whole blood is not recommended and platelet function deteriorates rapidly in stored whole blood.

## 2.87 Answers

A **False** – Prednisolone crosses the placenta. Fetal complications include neonatal adrenal insufficiency and thymic hypoplasia – unlikely to occur if the dose is <15 mg/day.

B **True** – Azathioprine is teratogenic in animals but not humans. Crosses the placenta but the fetal liver cannot convert it to its active form, 6-mercaptopurine. Associated with SGA babies and dose-related myelosuppression in the fetus.

C **False.**

D **False** – Tacrolimus crosses the placenta and is associated with hyperkalaemia and renal insufficiency.

Note:

- Cyclosporine is not teratogenic but is associated with SGA babies.
- Insufficient data are available on the use of mycophenolate mofetil and sirolimus.

## 2.88 Answers

A **False** – Augmentin is not licensed for use in pregnancy. Given the results of the ORACLE trial, it should be avoided in pregnancy.

B **False.**

C **True** – Warfarin is absolutely contraindicated because heparin is safer.

D **False.**

## 2.89 Answers

A **False** – Lithium is not absolutely contraindicated although it is teratogenic.

B **False.**

C **False.**

D **False.**

Note:

- Very few drugs are absolutely contraindicated in pregnancy – a balance has to be struck between the risks and benefits and the availability of safer alternatives: compare warfarin and lithium.

## 2.90 Answers

**A** False.

**B** False.

**C** True – Causes purgation.

**D** True – Risk of toxicity – hypotonia.

Note:
- No drug is absolutely contraindicated in breastfeeding – need to balance potential risks and benefits, and the availability of alternative therapies.
- The only drugs known to carry a serious risk of harming the breastfed baby are antithyroid agents. The concentration of propylthiouracil may be higher in milk than in maternal plasma. Also note:
  1. Aspirin – Possible risk of Reye's syndrome.
  2. Carbimazole – May affect neonatal thyroid function, nodular goiter; avoid.
  3. Nalidixic acid – Can cause haemolytic anaemia.
  4. Propylthiouracil – Risk of hypothyroidism/agranulocytosis/nodular goiter; avoid.
  5. Tetracyclines – Possibility of dental discolouration.

## 2.91 Answers

**A** True – Aspirin is a prostaglandin synthase inhibitor.

**B** True – Present in breast milk and may cause Reye's syndrome in the neonate.

**C** True – Low-dose aspirin and calcium supplementation appear to reduce the risks of hypertension in pregnancy and of pre-eclampsia, especially in women at high risk.

**D** False.

Note:
- Associated with premature closure of the ductus arteriosus, pulmonary hypertension in the neonate and oligohydramnios.
- Large doses may cause haemorrhagic complications in the mother and fetus.

## 2.92 Answers

**A** True – Major anomalies include heart defects, cleft lip or palate, skeletal malformations and microcephaly, IUGR and learning disability.

**B** True – Minor malformations include strabismus, hypertelorism, distal digital hypoplasia, nail hypoplasia, clubfoot, broad nasal bridge and abnormal dermatoglyphic patterns.

**C** False.

**D** True – See B.

## 2.93 Answers

**A** **True** – Most common features are nasal hypoplasia and stippled epiphyses/malformed vertebral bodies.

**B** **True** – Other features include hydrocephalus, microcephaly, IUGR, eye abnormalities and postnatal developmental delay.

**C** **True.**

**D** **False.**

Note:
- Warfarin embryopathy occurs in 15–25% of pregnancies when used in the first trimester.

## 2.94 Answers

**A** **True** – Chondrodysplasia punctata (stippled epiphyses, malformed vertebral bodies, nasal hypoplasia), microcephaly, hydrocephalus, IUGR, congenital cataract, asplenia syndrome, diaphragmatic hernia. Fetal intracerebral and retroplacental haemorrhages.

**B** **True** – Dysmorphic facies, cleft lip/palate, hypertelorism, broad nasal bridge, hypoplasia of the distal phalanges, nail hypoplasia, IUGR, learning disability.

**C** **False** – Heparin does not cross the placenta.

**D** **False** – Immunosupressive agents such as cyclosporine and azathioprine are not teratogenic but may be associated with low birth weight.

## 2.95 Answers

**A** **True** – Complications of sickle cell disease are more common in pregnancy and ~35% of pregnancies will develop crises.

**B** **False.**

**C** **True** – Atrial or ventricular septal defect with pulmonary hypertension and right-to-left shunt. Cyanotic heart disease with ~50% mortality in pregnancy.

**D** **False** – Multiple sclerosis is less likely to present for the first time and is less likely to relapse during pregnancy.

### 2.96 Answers

**A** **True** – Intravenous gamma-globulin may be used in resistant cases. IgG may cross the placenta and cause fetal thrombocytopenia – fetal risks are, however, small.

**B** **False** – Splenectomy should be avoided in pregnancy.

**C** **False.**

**D** **False** – Corticosteroids are first-line treatment.

Note:

- Immune thrombocytopenia affects 1–2:10 000 pregnancies.
- Auto-antibodies against platelet surface antigens cause platelet destruction by the reticuloendothelial system.
- Diagnosis is one of exclusion after other causes of thrombocytopenia have been ruled out. Specialized labs may measure antiplatelet antibodies.
- Course of disease is not affected by pregnancy.
- Platelet transfusion for bleeding or to cover labour/surgery if platelet count $<80 \times 10^9$/L.

### 2.97 Answers

**A** **False.**

**B** **False.**

**C** **False** – Iron overload is not a complication of massive blood transfusion as this is undertaken to replace severe blood loss. Iron overload occurs after recurrent blood transfusion to treat haemoglobinopathies.

**D** **False** – *Hyper*kalaemia from high potassium in stored cells

Note:

- Recognized complications are: thrombocytopaenia and coagulopathy due to depleted clotting factors, hypocalcaemia and hyperkalaemia.

# 3. Oncology: Questions

**3.1**   Ovarian teratomas:

A Typically present in the fifth decade of life.
B 50% are bilateral.
C The presence of immature neural tissue is of prognostic significance.
D AFP levels are typically elevated.

**3.2**   Benign cystic teratoma of the ovary:

A Are associated with menorrhagia.
B Are more likely to rupture during pregnancy.
C Are multilocular.
D Are lined by squamous epithelium.

**3.3**   Ovarian thecomas:

A Are typically benign.
B Are typically bilateral.
C Characteristically occur before puberty.
D Are characteristically associated with endometrial hyperplasia.

**3.4**   Ovarian thecomas:

A Are associated with Meig's syndrome.
B Are associated with virilization.
C Typically produce oestrogen.
D Characteristically have a high degree of cellular atypia.

**3.5**   The following are components of Meig's syndrome:

A Amenorrhoea.
B Pelvic mass.
C Ascites.
D Pericardial effusion.

**3.6**   Dysgerminomas:

A  Are derived from the sex cords.
B  Are associated with gonadal dysgenesis.
C  50% are bilateral.
D  Are typically radiosensitive.

**3.7**   Ovarian dysgerminomas:

A  Have a peak incidence in women under the age of 30 years.
B  Are associated with hirsutism.
C  Are characteristically bilateral.
D  Are typically radiosensitive.

**3.8**   Ovarian dysgerminomas:

A  Show lymphoid infiltration of the fibrous stroma on
   histological examination.
B  Are associated with elevated serum inhibin-A concentration.
C  Typically spread to the omentum rather than the para-aortic
   nodes.
D  Characteristically occur in women with Turner's syndrome.

**3.9**   Granulosa cell tumours of the ovary:

A  Typically lead to recurrence within 2 years of diagnosis.
B  Are bilateral in over 20% of cases.
C  Can occur at any age.
D  Typically present with stage IV disease.

**3.10**   Granulosa cell tumours of the ovary:

A  Are typically chemosensitive.
B  Should be managed with conservative surgery in young women.
C  Typically present with stage III disease.
D  With appropriate treatment have a 5-year survival of 40%.

**3.11**   Oestrogen-secreting ovarian tumours include:

A  Endometriomata.
B  Dysgerminomas.
C  Granulosa cell tumours.
D  Serous cystadenoma.

**3.12** CA-125 levels are elevated (>35 U/ml) in the following conditions:

A Ovarian granulosa cell tumours.
B Endometriosis.
C Uterine fibroids.
D Normal pregnancy.

**3.13** The following tumour markers are useful in monitoring the ovarian tumours listed:

A AFP – yolk sac tumours.
B Oestrogen – granulosa cell tumours.
C HCG – ovarian choriocarcinoma.
D Thyroxine – ovarian teratoma, struma ovarii.

**3.14** Carcinoembryonic antigen:

A Is more likely to be elevated in women with mucinous compared to serous ovarian cancers.
B Is more likely to be elevated in undifferentiated compared to well differentiated tumours.
C Is elevated in women with endometriosis.
D Is elevated in women with large uterine fibroids.

**3.15** The risk of ovarian cancer:

A Is increased in nulliparous women.
B Is increased in women with one first-degree relative with ovarian cancer.
C Is increased in women with blood group A.
D Is lower in women with blood group O.

**3.16** In a woman with a family history of ovarian cancer:

A A single first-degree relative with ovarian cancer is associated with a 10-fold increase in risk of ovarian cancer.
B A family history of colorectal and prostate cancer is suggestive of the Lynch I syndrome.
C Hysterectomy with ovarian conservation is associated with a reduction in ovarian cancer risk.
D Prophylactic oophorectomy eliminates the risk of ovarian cancer.

**3.17** With respect to mutations in the BRCA1 and BRCA2 genes:

A The BRCA1 gene is located on chromosome 17.

B Mutations in the BRCA2 gene are associated with a 7% life-time risk of breast cancer in male carriers.

C Mutations in the BRCA1 gene are associated with a 30% life-time risk of breast cancer in male carriers.

D BRCA1 and BRCA2 mutations are associated with an 80–90% life-time risk of breast cancer in women.

**3.18** With respect to pregnancy and breast cancer:

A Full-term pregnancy is associated with an increase in breast cancer risk which persists for 3–4 years.

B Women who develop breast cancer during pregnancy have a better prognosis.

C Pregnancy after treatment for breast cancer does not significantly alter prognosis.

D A delay of 2–3 years is recommended between treatment for breast cancer and subsequent pregnancy.

**3.19** With respect to the risk of malignancy index for ovarian cysts:

A Women with a risk of malignancy index of 20 are at high risk of ovarian cancer.

B The presence of ascites is used in deriving the ultrasound score.

C A unilateral multilocular cyst with no solid areas and no evidence of ascites or metastases should be assigned an ultrasound score of 5.

D A 60-year-old post-menopausal woman with a 4-cm simple unilateral ovarian cyst and a normal CA-125 level may be managed conservatively.

**3.20** With respect to epithelial ovarian cancer in the UK:

A It causes more deaths than any other genital tract cancer.

B There is an association with prolonged use of the COCP.

C 5-year survival is higher with serous compared to mucinous adenocarcinomas.

D Second-look laparotomy is associated with improved 5-year survival.

**3.21** With respect to epithelial ovarian cancer in the UK:

A There is an association with high parity.
B There is an association with primary breast cancer.
C Chemotherapy is recommended for borderline tumours.
D Bowel resection is not justifiable.

**3.22** The following stagings of carcinoma of the ovary are accurate:

A Stage Ia – tumour confined to one ovary with intact capsule and no ascites.
B Stage Ic – tumour confined to the ovaries with positive peritoneal cytology.
C Stage IV – intrahepatic metastases.
D Stage IIb – palpable retroperitoneal lymph nodes.

**3.23** With respect to the FIGO staging of ovarian cancer:

A Stage II tumours are limited to the ovaries.
B Secondary deposits in the omentum indicate stage III disease.
C Ascites can be present in stage I disease.
D A pleural effusion with negative cytology indicates stage III disease.

**3.24** With respect to ovarian cancer:

A Primary tumours are characterized by the presence of signet-ring cells.
B Prognosis is improved by the instillation of cytotoxic agents into the peritoneal cavity at laparotomy.
C Dysgerminomas are histologically identical to seminomata of the testes.
D Dysgerminomas are highly radiosensitive.

**3.25** The following are prognostic factors in women with malignant epithelial ovarian tumours:

A Histological tumour type.
B Histological grade.
C Pre-operative tumour size.
D Size of residual disease after surgery.

3.26 In the treatment of a 40-year-old woman with ovarian carcinoma:

A Surgical treatment alone is recommended in well differentiated stage Ib tumours.
B Stage IV disease has a 25% 5-year survival.
C In the presence of a pleural effusion, primary chemotherapy rather than surgery should be recommended.
D Postoperative adjuvant chemotherapy should be recommended for stage Ic disease.

3.27 With respect to epithelial ovarian cancer in the UK:

A Infracolic omentectomy should be performed in stage II disease.
B Second-line chemotherapy often produces dramatic remission.
C Bowel resection is not justifiable.
D Chemotherapy is not indicated for stage I disease.

3.28 Borderline epithelial ovarian tumours:

A Are diagnosed on clinical examination.
B Can be diagnosed by measuring serum concentration of tumour markers.
C Can be diagnosed on CT scan.
D May be associated with invasive implants, which carry a worse prognosis.

3.29 The following are recognized side effects of paclitaxel:

A Bradycardia.
B Loss of eyebrows and axillary hair.
C Hypersensitivity.
D Neutropaenia.

3.30 Paclitaxel:

A Is usually administered orally.
B Is usually administered in conjunction with corticosteroids and H1 and H2 antagonists.
C Causes hair loss in most patients which involves eyebrows, pubic and axillary hair.
D Is excreted principally by the kidneys.

**3.31** With respect to chemotherapeutic agents used in gynaecological oncology:

A  Cisplatin is more nephrotoxic than carboplatin.
B  Cisplatin causes less nausea and vomiting than carboplatin.
C  Forced diuresis is usually employed during paclitaxel therapy.
D  Intestinal perforation is a recognized complication of methotrexate.

**3.32** The following drugs are associated with the listed side effect:

A  Cyclophosphamide – hypomagnesaemia.
B  Cisplatin – haemorrhagic cystitis.
C  Paclitaxel – severe nausea and vomiting.
D  Paclitaxel – high-frequency hearing loss.

**3.33** During chemotherapy for gynaecological malignancies:

A  Administration of N-acetylcystine or mesna reduces the risk of haemorrhagic cystitis associated with cyclophosphamide.
B  Corticosteroids significantly reduce the risk of nausea and vomiting.
C  Forced diuresis reduces the risk of renal toxicity associated with cisplatin.
D  Methotrexate toxicity is worsened by concurrent administration of aspirin.

**3.34** Doxorubicin hydrochloride (adriamycin):

A  Is an antibiotic.
B  Is an antimetabolite.
C  Is cardiotoxic.
D  Is the drug of choice in the treatment of adenocarcinoma of the cervix.

**3.35** The following are associated with an increased risk of endometrial cancer:

A  Nulliparity.
B  Use of the combined oral contraceptive pill.
C  Family history of cervical cancer.
D  Polycystic ovary syndrome.

**3.36** The following are associated with an increased risk of developing endometrial cancer:

A Late menopause.
B Personal history of breast cancer.
C Use of raloxifen.
D Use of tamoxifen.

**3.37** The risk of endometrial cancer is increased in:

A Women with a history of recurrent miscarriage.
B Women with a granulosa cell tumour.
C Women with an early menopause.
D Women on immunosuppressive therapy.

**3.38** The risk of endometrial cancer is increased in:

A Women who have never had a cervical smear.
B Nulliparous women.
C Women with diabetes mellitus.
D Women on tamoxifen.

**3.39** With respect to endometrial cancer:

A 15% of patients are <40 years of age.
B The median age at presentation is 75 years.
C The overall crude 5-year survival in the UK is ~85%.
D Serous carcinoma is the commonest histological type.

**3.40** With respect to endometrial hyperplasia:

A Simple hyperplasia is typically associated with endometrial carcinoma.
B Atypical hyperplasia carries a 1% risk of progression to endometrial carcinoma.
C There is an association with adjuvant tamoxifen use in women with breast cancer.
D Progesterone therapy is recommended in a 59-year-old woman with atypical hyperplasia.

3.41 With respect to the spread of endometrial carcinoma:

A ~50% of women with nodal disease have involvement of the para-aortic nodes.

B Spread to pelvic nodes occurs more commonly than in cervical cancer.

C There is an association between the depth of myometrial invasion and the presence of nodal metastases.

D Spread to the ovary is uncommon in women with metastatic disease.

3.42 With respect to post-menopausal bleeding:

A The risk of endometrial cancer increases with age.

B The incidence is higher at age 80 compared to 50 years.

C Endometrial carcinoma is the commonest cause.

D Carcinoma of the vulva is a recognized cause.

3.43 With respect to staging of endometrial cancer:

A Stage Ia – tumour confined to the myometrium.

B Stage IIIa – positive peritoneal cytology.

C Stage IV – invasion of bladder or bowel mucosa.

D Stage IV – involvement of inguinal nodes.

3.44 A 65-year-old woman with post-menopausal bleeding is found to have an endometrial carcinoma on biopsy with involvement of endocervical stroma on MRI imaging:

A These findings are consistent with a stage IIb tumour.

B Radical abdominal hysterectomy with bilateral salpingo-oophrectomy and pelvic lymphadenectomy is the recommended operation.

C Postoperative adjuvant chemotherapy would be recommended if the MRI findings are confirmed histologically.

D The 5-year survival is ~20%.

3.45 Endometrial hyperplasia is characteristically associated with:

A Anovulatory cycles.

B Hyperthyroidism.

C Vaginal adenosis.

D Hyperprolactinaemia.

**3.46** Endometrial hyperplasia is characteristically associated with:

A The use of IUCD.
B Essential hypertension.
C Prolonged post-partum anovulation.
D Cushing's syndrome.

**3.47** Characteristic features of atypical endometrial hyperplasia include:

A Secretory changes in the endometrium.
B Ovulatory cycles.
C Hirsutism.
D Premenstrual tension.

**3.48** Characteristic features of atypical endometrial hyperplasia include:

A Association with uterine fibroids.
B Foci of squamous metaplasia.
C A loss of nuclear polarization in the epithelium.
D Enlarged nucleoli.

**3.49** Endometrial carcinoma:

A Is histologically well differentiated in the majority of cases.
B At the time of diagnosis, has metastasized to the ovary in 30% of women.
C 50% of women present with stage I disease.
D Positive peritoneal cytology is present in 1% of patients.

**3.50** Endometrial carcinoma:

A Metastasizes typically to the supraclavicular node.
B Has a better prognosis when it occurs in women below the age of 45 years.
C Has a 10% 5-year survival rate for stage IV disease.
D Is more likely to recur in women with positive peritoneal cytology than in those in whom cytology is negative.

**3.51** Endometrial carcinoma:

A Typically presents with intermenstrual bleeding.
B Is a sequel to prenatal oestrogen treatment.
C Is associated with use of the COCP for more than 10 years.
D May involve the para-aortic nodes without pelvic node involvement.

3.52   Adenocarcinoma of the uterus:

A Metastasizes characteristically to the supraclavicular lymph nodes.
B Uterine size is a reliable prognostic indicator.
C In stage I disease, the incidence of pelvic lymph node metastases is about 3%.
D Pre-operative treatment with progestogens significantly improves prognosis.

3.53   Endometrial cancer typically metastasizes to:

A The brain.
B Pouch of Douglas.
C Para-aortic lymph nodes.
D Lungs.

3.54   Endometrial cancer typically metastasizes to:

A Liver.
B Ovaries.
C Cervix.
D Inguinal nodes.

3.55   The following are associated with an increase in the risk of long-term complications from radiotherapy for cervical cancer:

A Obesity.
B PID.
C Severe vascular disease.
D Previous abdominal surgery.

3.56   The following are associated with an increase in the risk of long-term complications from radiotherapy for cervical cancer:

A Previous pelvic surgery.
B Weight loss.
C Use of intracavitary therapy only.
D Use of hyperbaric oxygen.

3.57 With respect to Lichen sclerosus:

A Excision of affected vulval skin is recognized treatment.
B $CO_2$ laser vaporization is recognized treatment.
C There is an association with squamous cell cercinoma of the vulva.
D There is an association with HPV infection.

3.58 Lichen planus:

A Involves the oral mucosa and gum margins.
B Involves the vagina.
C Topical oestrogen is the recognized treatment.
D May require treatment with systemic steroids or azathioprine.

3.59 With respect to the vulva:

A Paget's disease is associated with apocrine carcinoma.
B Lichen sclerosus should be treated with simple vulvectomy.
C Pruritus is a feature of VIN3.
D Adenocarcinoma accounts for 25% of vulval malignancies.

3.60 Recognized causes of granulomatous lesions of the vulva include:

A Paget's disease.
B Lichen sclerosus.
C Behçet's syndrome.
D Crohn's disease.

3.61 The following conditions of the gastrointestinal tract may also affect the vulva:

A Crohn's disease.
B Ulcerative colitis.
C Diverticular disease.
D Coeliac disease.

3.62 Non-cystic lesions of the vulva include:

A Bartholin.
B Nabothian cyst.
C Accessory breast tissue.
D Hydradenoma.

**3.63** Paget's disease of the vulva:

    A Typically occurs in post-menopausal women.
    B Is associated with an underlying squamous cell carcinoma.
    C Involving the perianal area is associated with adenocarcinoma of the rectum.
    D Is characterized histologically by the presence of Call-Exner bodies.

**3.64** Vulval intraepithelial neoplasia:

    A Typically presents with vulval itching.
    B Is associated with immunosuppression.
    C Spontaneous regression may occur.
    D Can be treated by $CO_2$ laser vaporization.

**3.65** The following are associated with an increased risk of vulval carcinoma:

    A Obesity.
    B Diabetes mellitus.
    C Early menopause.
    D Nulliparity.

**3.66** Squamous cell carcinoma of the vulva:

    A Make up 60% of malignant vulval tumours.
    B Typically spread to the superficial and deep inguinal nodes.
    C Stage Ia tumours are confined to the vulva with <1 mm depth of invasion.
    D Stage Ib tumours are <2 cm in diameter with no clinically suspicious nodes.

**3.67** With respect to staging of vulval cancer:

    A Stage III – tumour extending beyond the vulva without grossly positive groin nodes.
    B Stage III – tumour confined to the vulva with suspicious groin nodes.
    C Stage IV – involvement of the urethra.
    D Stage IV – involvement of bladder mucosa.

**3.68** The following complications are associated with surgical treatment of vulval carcinoma:

A Wound breakdown.
B Venous thromboembolism.
C Lymphoedema.
D Lymphocysts.

**3.69** With respect to carcinoma of the vagina:

A The majority of primary tumours are adenocarcinomas.
B Stage I tumours are confined to the vaginal wall.
C Stage III tumours involve the pelvic side-wall.
D Stage IIa tumours involve the parametrium.

**3.70** Clear cell adenocarcinoma of the vagina:

A Typically presents in post-menopausal women.
B Is associated with in utero exposure to diethylstilboestrol.
C Should be treated by chemotherapy.
D Is associated with true gonadal dysgenesis.

**3.71** Primary carcinoma of the fallopian tube:

A Is bilateral in about 70% of cases.
B Is typically radiosensitive.
C Presents with profuse watery vaginal discharge.
D Has a peak incidence in the sixth decade of life.

**3.72** Primary carcinoma of the fallopian tube:

A Is usually a squamous cell carcinoma.
B Has a 10% 5-year survival rate.
C Typically presents with ascites.
D Is associated with elevated CA-125 levels.

## 3.1 Answers

**A** **False** – Median age at presentation is 30 years.

**B** **False** – Dermoid cysts are bilateral in 10% of cases; immature teratomas are typically unilateral.

**C** **True** – Immature teratomas have a variable amount of immature tissue, usually of neuroectodermal origin. May also contain areas of yolk sac tumour or choriocarcinoma, which produce AFP and HCG, respectively. The amount of immature tissue, degree of atypia and mitotic activity correlate with prognosis.

**D** **False.**

## 3.2 Answers

**A** **False.**

**B** **True.**

**C** **False** – Usually unilocular cysts <15 cm with ectodermal structures.

**D** **True** – Lined with epidermis and contain skin appendages.

Note:
- Dermoid cysts (mature cystic teratoma) account for 40% of all ovarian neoplasms.
- Dermoid cysts may contain endodermal derivatives such as thyroid tissue which is present in 5–20% of tumours.
- Majority (60%) are asymptomatic, 3.5–10% undergo torsion, <5% rupture spontaneously.
- 2% may contain malignant components – usually squamous cell carcinoma.
- Immature teratomas account for 1% of all ovarian teratomas. Solid tumours are usually malignant.

## 3.3 Answers

**A** **True** – Benign solid lobulated tumours.

**B** **False.**

**C** **False.**

**D** **False.**

Note:
- Thecomas are less likely to rupture than granulosa cell tumours.
- Fibromas with >3 mitoses per 10 high-power fields are considered fibrosarcomas.

## 3.4 Answers

**A** **True** – May be associated with Meig's syndrome (pelvic mass, ascites and pleural effusion, usually right sided).

**B** **False.**

**C** **False** – Thecomas may be hormonally active and produce oestrogen with a presentation similar to that described for granulosa tumours – such tumours usually have a granulosa-cell element which may be malignant.

**D** **False.**

## 3.5 Answers

**A** False.
**B** True.
**C** True.
**D** False.

Note: See 3.4A.

## 3.6 Answers

**A** False.
**B** True.
**C** **False** – 10–15% are bilateral.
**D** **True** – Exquisitely radiosensitive.

Note:
- Commonest malignant germ cell tumour and make up 2–5% of malignant ovarian tumours.
- Solid tumours which typically present with abdominal mass or pressure symptoms.
- No reliable serum marker.
- 70% present with stage I disease.
- Analogous to the seminoma in males.
- Associated with gonadal dysgenesis and karyotype is recommended, especially in an amenorrhoeic woman.
- Histology: groups of large round tumour cells separated by fibrous tissue septae infiltrated by lymphocytes. Minimal lymphocytic response is associated with poor prognosis.

## 3.7 Answers

**A** **True** – 90% occur in young women <30 years.
**B** False.
**C** **False** – 10–15% are bilateral.
**D** **True** – Exquisitely radiosensitive.

## 3.8 Answers

**A** True.
**B** False.
**C** **False** – Lymphatic spread to the para-aortic nodes is more common than surface intraperitoneal metastases.
**D** False.

## 3.9 Answers

**A** False.
**B** **False** – 5% are bilateral.
**C** **True** – 5% occur in pre-pubertal girls, 50% occur in post-menopausal women.
**D** **False** – 85–90% present with stage I disease.

## 3.10 Answers

**A** **False.**

**B** **False** – Radical surgery should be recommended, even in young women with stage Ia disease because of high risk of recurrence.

**C** **False** – See 3.9D.

**D** **False** – With radical surgery, 5-, 10- and 20-year survival = 94%, 82% and 62%, respectively.

Note:

- ~2% of all ovarian tumours.
- Produce oestrogen.
- Present with isosexual precocious puberty, menorrhagia and irregular bleeding, post-menopausal bleeding or acute abdominal pain because of their tendency to rupture.
- Adjuvant therapy has not been shown to be of value.

## 3.11 Answers

**A** **False.**

**B** **False.**

**C** **True** – Granulosa cell tumours are the only oestrogen-secreting ovarian tumours. Thecomas may secrete oestrogen but these tumours usually contain a granulose-cell element which may be malignant.

**D** **False.**

## 3.12 Answers

**A** **False.**

**B** **True.**

**C** **True.**

**D** **True.**

Note:

- Normal: CA-125 <35 U/ml.
- Increased:
  1. CA-125 >35 highly correlated with cancer.
  2. CA-125 >65 associated with cancer in 90% pelvic mass.
  3. CA-125 >200 unlikely to be due to benign condition.
- Normal in 50% of stage I ovarian cancer.
- Increased in 85% of ovarian cancer overall.
- Non-malignant causes of increased CA-125: endometriosis, pelvic inflammatory disease, uterine fibroids, pregnancy, liver cirrhosis, post-menopause, tuberculous peritonitis, pelvic irradiation.
- Malignant causes of increased CA-125: ovarian cancer, liver cancer, lung cancer, breast cancer, colon cancer, pancreatic cancer, endometrial cancer, cervical cancer.

## 3.13 Answers

**A** **True** – Yolk sac (endodermal sinus) tumours produce AFP.

**B** **True** – Granulosa cell tumours produce oestrogen and are associated with PMB or precocious puberty.

**C** **True** – Choriocarcinomas produce HCG.

**D** **True** – Struma ovarii produce thyroxine.

## 3.14 Answers

**A True** – CEA is elevated most often in mucinous cystadenocarcinomas.
**B True** – Levels are higher in poorly differentiated tumours.
**C False** – Not elevated in fibroids or endometriosis (CA-125 elevated).
**D False.**

## 3.15 Answers

**A True** – Reproductive history is associated with increased risk: early menarche, late menopause, nulliparity or having first pregnancy after the age of 30.
**B True** – Family history is associated with increased risk: ovarian cancer, breast cancer, or colorectal cancer. About 10% of ovarian cancers are hereditary, mainly associated with BRCA1 and BRCA2.
**C True.**
**D True.**

Note:

- Increased risk also seen with: age – most ovarian cancers develop after menopause; obesity - the risk is increased by 50% in the heaviest women; fertility drugs – may be associated with small increase in risk; personal history of breast cancer.
- Decreased risk seen with: long-term use of COCP; tubal ligation; multiparity; breastfeeding; especially for >1 year; blood group O.

## 3.16 Answers

**A False** – The risk of ovarian cancer in first- and second-degree relatives of women with ovarian cancer is increased 3.6- and 2.9-fold, respectively, compared to women without a family history.
**B False** – Lynch I syndrome – site-specific colorectal cancer. Lynch II syndrome – autosomal dominant predisposition to colorectal cancer in addition to endometrial, ovarian, stomach, pancreatic, renal tract and small bowel cancers.
**C True.**
**D False** – Prophylactic oophorectomy reduces but does not eliminate the risk of ovarian cancer and primary peritoneal carcinomatosis may still occur.

Note:

- A family history of pre-menopausal breast cancer is associated with a ~50% increase in the risk of developing ovarian cancer.
- A family history of ovarian cancer, however, is not associated with an increased risk of developing breast cancer.

### 3.17 Answers

A **True** – Thought to be a tumour suppressor gene located on 17q21.

B **True.**

C **False** – Not associated with breast cancer in males.

D **True** – The cumulative risk of developing breast cancer by the age of 70 years is 80–90% in BRCA1 mutation carriers, the risk of developing ovarian cancer being 30–60%. Risk of developing breast cancer by the age of 70 years is 80–90% in BRCA2 mutation carriers, whereas the risk of developing ovarian cancer is 15–20%.

Note:

* BRCA1 germline mutations are thought to be responsible for 90% of hereditary ovarian cancers and 50% of hereditary breast cancers. Carrier rate in the general population ~1:800.
* BRCA2 gene is located on 13q12.
* BRCA2 germline mutations are thought to be responsible for 40% of hereditary breast cancers and 5–10% of hereditary ovarian cancers.

### 3.18 Answers

A **True** – Full-term pregnancy is associated with an increased risk of breast cancer (relative risk 1.21) which is maximum 3-4 years after delivery followed by a subsequent decline.

B **False** – Women who develop breast cancer during or soon after pregnancy have a worse prognosis, probably related to difficulty and delay in diagnosis.

C **True** – In women who become pregnant after treatment for breast cancer, the prognosis is unaffected.

D **True** – A delay of at least 2 years is recommended before pregnancy in women treated for breast cancer.

Note:

* Breastfeeding is not contraindicated in women who have had conservative surgery + radiotherapy for breast cancer.

### 3.19 Answers

A **False** – RMI <25 = low risk with <3% risk of cancer; RMI 25–250 = moderate risk with a 20% risk of cancer; RMI >250 = high risk with a 75% risk of cancer.

B **True.**

C **False.**

D **True.**

Note:

* The risk of malignancy index (RMI) is an effective way of triaging women into low, moderate or high risk of malignancy for management by general gynaecologists, cancer units or cancer centres, respectively.
* RMI = U x M x CA-125:
    1. U = Ultrasound score – one point for each of the following: multilocular cysts, evidence of solid areas, evidence of metastases, presence of ascites, bilateral lesions. U = 0 for score of 0; U = 1 for score of 1, U = 3 for score of 3–5.
    2. M = Menopausal score, 1 for pre- and 3 for post-menopausal.
    3. CA-125 level in U/ml.

### 3.20 Answers

**A** **True** – Causes more deaths than any other gynaecological cancer. Life-time risk by age 65 years = 0.9%; overall life-time risk = 2.1% (1 in 48).

**B** **False** – Prolonged use of COCP is protective.

**C** **False** – Stage-for-stage, there is no difference in mortality with different epithelial types; histological type is not of prognostic significance.

**D** **False** – Second-look laparotomy has not been shown to be associated with improved survival.

### 3.21 Answers

**A** **False** – Parity is protective.

**B** **True** – A personal history of primary breast cancer is associated with increased risk of ovarian cancer.

**C** **False** – Chemotherapy is not recommended for borderline tumours and does not improve prognosis.

**D** **False** – Bowel resection may be required during primary cytoreductive surgery although morbidity associated with multiple/extensive resection should be considered.

### 3.22 Answers

**A** **True** – Stage I - limited to the ovaries: Ia - one ovary, capsule intact, no ascites; Ib - both ovaries, capsules intact, no ascites; Ic – capsule breached or ascites.

**B** **True** – See A.

**C** **True** – Stage IV – distant/intrahepatic metastases.

**D** **False** – Stage II – presence of peritoneal deposits in pelvis: IIa – on uterus or tubes; IIb – on other pelvic organs; IIc – with ascites.

### 3.23 Answers

**A** **False** – See 3.22 D.

**B** **True** – Stage III - peritoneal deposits outside pelvis.

**C** **True** – See 3.22 A.

**D** **False.**

Note:

- Stage Ia treatment – surgery. 80% 5-year survival rate.
- Stage II treatment – surgery then chemotherapy. 60% 5-year survival rate.
- Stage III treatment – surgery then chemotherapy. 25% 5-year survival rate.
- Stage IV treatment – surgery for palliation only, then chemotherapy. 5–10% 5-year survival rate.

**3.24** **Answers**

**A** **False** – Signet ring cells occur in Krukenberg tumours, which are secondary.
**B** **False** – No evidence that intraperitoneal instillation of cytotoxic agents at laparotomy improves prognosis.
**C** **True** – Dysgerminomas are analogous to the seminoma in males.
**D** **True** – Originate in germ cells and are radiosensitive.

**3.25** **Answers**

**A** **False** – Histological type, adhesions, extracapsular growth and size of tumour are not of prognostic significance.
**B** **True** – Degree of differentiation (grade) most important factor in stage I disease.
**C** **False.**
**D** **True** – Size of residual disease after surgery – women with no/minimal disease.

Note:
- Rupture before and during surgery are poor prognostic indicators for stage I disease.
- Young age is associated with better prognosis.

**3.26** **Answers**

**A** **True** – For well differentiated stage Ib tumour, adjuvant chemotherapy is not recommended - no effect on overall survival or disease-free survival.
**B** **False** – Stage IV disease: 5–10% 5-year survival.
**C** **False** – In women with ovarian cancer, pleural effusion may be non-malignant. Presence of malignant pleural effusion = stage IV disease.
**D** **True** – For stage Ic or poorly differentiated stage Ib disease, adjuvant chemotherapy is recommended.

**3.27** **Answers**

**A** **True** – The operation of choice is TAH + BSO + omentectomy.
**B** **False** – The response from second-line chemotherapy after relapse is usually disappointing.
**C** **False** – Bowel resection may be required although morbidity associated with multiple/extensive resection should be considered.
**D** **False** – Primary chemotherapy is usually recommended for stage Ib and beyond.

### 3.28 Answers

**A False** – Diagnosis is made on histological examination, which may be difficult, especially in mucinous tumours.

**B False.**

**C False.**

**D True** – Invasive implants may be present and are associated with poorer prognosis.

Note:
- Borderline epithelial ovarian tumours account for about 10% of all epithelial tumours of the ovary, of which 30% are mucinous.
- Varying degree of nuclear atypia, increased mitotic activity with multilayering and cellular buds but no invasion.
- Peritoneal and omental lesions may be present – some may regress after removal of the primary.
- Chemotherapy is not indicated as it does not improve prognosis.

### 3.29 Answers

**A True** – Side effects include asymptomatic bradycardia during administration and other more serious bradyarrhythmias, including heart block; mucositis and sensory peripheral neuropathy.

**B True** – Alopecia is almost universal and involves all body hair sites including eyebrows, pubic and axillary hair.

**C True** – Associated with hypersensitivity reactions – risk reduced by pre-treatment with corticosteroids, H1 and H2 antagonists.

**D True** – Principal toxicity is neutropaenia. Onset 8–10 days after administration with complete recovery by 15–21 days.

### 3.30 Answers

**A False** – Administered by slow intravenous infusion over 3–24 hours.

**B True.**

**C True** – See 3.29 B.

**D False** - Metabolized by hepatic cytochrome P450-dependent pathways. 5–10% excreted by the kidneys.

Note:
- Paclitaxel is 95% protein bound.
- Hepatic enzyme inducers accelerate paclitaxel metabolism.
- In combination chemotherapy with platinum agents, paclitaxel should be administered first as this reduces risk of myelotoxicity.

## 3.31 Answers

**A** **True** – Carboplatin causes less renal or oto-toxicity.

**B** **False** – Carboplatin causes less nausea and vomiting.

**C** **False** – Platinum agents are direct renal tubular toxins and renal damage is the major dose-limiting toxicity and is associated with hypomagnesaemia. Renal damage can be reduced by forced diuresis using saline or mannitol or by administration in hypertonic saline.

**D** **True** – Mucositis is a significant complication of methotrexate therapy with a risk of secondary infection or intestinal perforation.

## 3.32 Answers

**A** **False** – Associated with acute haemorrhagic cystitis (as is its analogue, ifosfamide).

**B** **False.**

**C** **False** – Very little tendency to cause nausea and vomiting. See 3.29 and 3.30.

**D** **False** – See 3.29 and 3.30.

## 3.33 Answers

**A** **True** – Cyclophosphamide is associated with acute haemorrhagic cystitis (as is its analogue ifosfamide). This can be prevented by maintaining high urine output or by the co-administration of N-acetylcysteine or mesna, which neutralize acrolein.

**B** **True** – Nausea and vomiting can be reduced by use of 5-HT antagonist ondansetron, H2 antagonists and corticosteroids.

**C** **True** – Cisplatin is a direct renal tubular toxin and renal damage is the major dose-limiting toxicity and is associated with hypomagnesaemia. Renal damage can be reduced by forced diuresis using saline or mannitol or by administration in hypertonic saline.

**D** **True** – Methotrexate is 50% protein bound and is excreted principally by the kidneys. Renal excretion is inhibited by the administration of weak organic acids such as aspirin and penicillin. Aspirin also displaces the drug from its binding sites, compounding toxicity.

## 3.34 Answers

**A** **True** – Doxorubicin is an antitumour antibiotic.

**B** **False** – Doxorubicin damages DNA by intercalation of the anthracycline portion, metal ion chelation, or by generation of free radicals. Also inhibits DNA topoisomerase II. Cytotoxic activity is cell cycle phase non-specific.

**C** **True** – Causes congestive cardiac failure and cardiomyopathy.

**D** **False** – Platinum agents are used in combination chemotherapy for cervical cancer.

Note:

- Doxorubicin is not absorbed orally.
- Metabolized by the liver and predominantly excreted in bile, 40–50% in faeces within 7 days.

### 3.35 Answers

A True.
B False.
C False.
D True.

Note:
- Increased risk of endometrial cancer is associated with: obesity, nulliparity, late menopause/early menarche, prolonged irregular bleeding, PCOS, unopposed oestrogen therapy or endogenous oestrogen from granulosa cell tumour, tamoxifen therapy, diabetes mellitus, hypertension, personal or family history of breast or colon cancer, high fat/low complex carbohydrate diet, sedentary lifestyle.
- Reduced risk is associated with COCP, physical exercise, smoking, late age at last birth, diet high in fruit and vegetables.

### 3.36 Answers

A True.
B True.
C False.
D True.

Note: See 3.35.

### 3.37 Answers

A False.
B True.
C False.
D False.

Note: See 3.35.

### 3.38 Answers

A False.
B True.
C True.
D True.

Note: See 3.35.

## 3.39 Answers

**A  False** – Incidence rises rapidly between the ages of 40 and 55 years and levels off after the menopause at about 44/100 000.

**B  False** – Median age at presentation is ~61 years.

**C  False** – 73% 5-year survival.

**D  False** – Endometroid adenocarcinoma is the commonest histological type.

Note:
- Risk of endometrial cancer by age 65 years = 0.6%. Overall life-time risk = 1.4% (1 in 73).
- ~25% increase in age-standardized incidence rates between 1991 and 2000 with ~1% increase in age-standardized mortality rates between 1993 and 2002.

## 3.40 Answers

**A  False** – Simple hyperplasia is increased volume of glandular tissue with marked variation in shape of glands with cystically dilated glands. Complex hyperplasia has more epithelial growth and there is glandular proliferation with glandular budding and reduction in stromal element. Back-to-back appearance of glands. ~2% risk of progression to carcinoma, 10% risk of progression to atypical hyperplasia.

**B  False** – Atypical hyperplasia is loss of nuclear polarization, enlarged rounded nuclei with hyperchromatism, enlarged nucleoli. Often associated with complex hyperplasia. ~50% risk of progression to carcinoma. An endometrial carcinoma may co-exist.

**C  True** – There is an increased risk in women on tamoxifen.

**D  False** – Atypical hyperplasia should be treated by hysterectomy.

## 3.41 Answers

**A  True** – 81% of women have no lymph node involvement at diagnosis. In 9% there is pelvic node involvement, in 7% pelvic and para-aortic node involvement, and in 3% para-aortic node involvement.

**B  False.**

**C  True.**

**D  False** – In women with metastatic disease, spread to the ovaries is common.

Note:
- Direct spread to the cervix.
- Direct metastatic spread to the para-aortic nodes without pelvic node involvement occurs. Supra-clavicular and inguinal nodes are rarely involved.
- Distant metastases are uncommon and only 2% present with stage IV disease.
- Positive peritoneal cytology present in 12–15% of patients, although in 50% of these, there is no histological evidence of extrauterine spread.

### 3.42   Answers

**A  True** – Risk of endometrial cancer increases with age in women with PMB: 5% below the age of 50 years, ~12% in 50–59 years age group, and over 30% in those over 70 years.

**B  False** – Incidence of PMB ~13% at age 50 years and ~0.2% at age 80 years.

**C  False** – Only ~10% of women with PMB have endometrial cancer and 66% have benign or non-neoplastic causes.

**D  True** – Malignant causes include carcinoma of the cervix (5.7%), vulva/vagina (1.4%), ovary (1.2%) and other malignancies (0.8%).

### 3.43   Answers

**A  False** – Ia – confined to the endometrium; Ib – <50% myometrial invasion; Ic – >50% myometrial invasion.

**B  True** – IIIa – invades serosa or adnexae or positive peritoneal cytology; IIIb – vaginal metastases; IIIc – pelvic or para-aortic nodes.

**C  True** – IVa – invades bladder or bowel mucosa; IVb – distant metastases, inguinal nodes.

**D  True** – See C.

Note:
- 80% present with stage I disease; 90% 5-year survival.
- Stage IIa – endocervical glandular involvement; IIb – endocervical stromal involvement. 10% present with stage II disease; 70% 5-year survival.
- 6% present with stage III disease; 40% 5-year survival.
- 2% present with stage IV disease; 25% 5-year survival.

### 3.44   Answers

**A  True** – Stage IIa – endocervical glands only; IIb – endocervical stroma involved.

**B  True** – Involvement of endocervical glands or stroma should be managed as for cervical cancer + BSO because of risk of adnexal involvement.

**C  False** – Post-op radiotherapy recommended for stage II disease.

**D  False** – 5-year survival for stage II disease is ~70%.

### 3.45   Answers

**A  True.**
**B  False.**
**C  False.**
**D  False.**

Note: See 3.35–3.38.

**3.46 Answers**

**A** False.
**B** True.
**C** False.
**D** False.

Note: See 3.35–3.38.

**3.47 Answers**

**A** False.
**B** False – Associated with anovulatory cycles.
**C** False.
**D** False.

Note:
- Characteristic features of atypical hyperplasia: loss of nuclear polarization, enlarged rounded nuclei with hyperchromatism, enlarged nucleoli. Often associated with complex hyperplasia. ~50% risk of progression to carcinoma. An endometrial carcinoma may co-exist.

**3.48 Answers**

**A** False.
**B** False – Squamous metaplasia is a feature of *adenoacanthoma* – endometrial adenocarcinoma with squamous metaplasia.
**C** True.
**D** True.

Note: See 3.47.

**3.49 Answers**

**A** False – Grade I – 29%, Grade II – 46%, Grade III – 24%. The majority are therefore moderately/poorly differentiated.
**B** False – Stage III – 6% of cases (adnexal involvement).
**C** False – Stage I – 80% of cases.
**D** False – Positive peritoneal cytology present in 12–15% of patients.

**3.50 Answers**

**A** False – See 3.41 A.
**B** True – Prognosis is better in younger women.
**C** False – 25% 5-year survival. 2% present with stage IV disease.
**D** True – Cases with positive lymph nodes or peritoneal cytology are more likely to recur than those without (50% versus 10%).

### 3.51 Answers

**A** **False** – Typically presents with PMB.
**B** **False** – Not associated with prenatal exposure to oestrogen.
**C** **False** – Prolonged use of COCP is protective.
**D** **True** – Direct metastatic spread to the para-aortic nodes without pelvic node involvement occurs. Supra-clavicular and inguinal nodes are rarely involved.

### 3.52 Answers

**A** **False** – 9.7% of women with clinical stage I disease and about 3% of those with histological stage I disease have positive lymph nodes. Lymph node metastasis is typically to the pelvic and para-aortic nodes.
**B** **False** – Tumour size, but not uterine size, is an important prognostic indicator.
**C** **True.**
**D** **False** – Progesterone pre-treatment does not improve outcome.

### 3.53 Answers

**A** **False.**
**B** **False.**
**C** **True** – Direct metastatic spread to the para-aortic nodes without pelvic node involvement occurs.
**D** **False.**

### 3.54 Answers

**A** **False.**
**B** **True** – In women with metastatic disease, spread to the ovaries is common.
**C** **False** – Direct spread to the cervix.
**D** **False** – Supraclavicular and inguinal nodes are rarely involved.

Note: See 3.41.

### 3.55 Answers

**A** **False.**
**B** **True** – Long-term complications are more likely in women with previous abdominal and pelvic surgery, PID, severe vascular disease, poor nutritional status and recent weight loss.
**C** **True.**
**D** **True.**

## 3.56 Answers

A **True.**
B **True.**
C **False.**
D **False** – There is no evidence that hyperbaric oxygen improves outcome.

Note: See 3.55B.

## 3.57 Answers

A **False** – Treat with topical corticosteroids such as clobetasol with nightly applications initially and then twice weekly once symptoms improve.
B **False.**
C **True** – Associated with a risk of squamous cell carcinoma of the vulva – 2.5–5% risk.
D **False.**

Note:
- Lichen sclerosis: thin, pearly-white skin with marked shrinkage and absorption of the labia minora and labial fusion to form a phimosis and narrow the intriotus that obscures the urethra. Fissuring may be present.
- Typically involves the perineum as a figure of 8 lesion encircling the vestibule and involving the clitoris, labia minora, inner aspect of labia majora and skin around the anus.
- Vagina, vestibule and anal canal are not involved.
- May also affect skin outside the perineum – trunk and limbs involved in 18%.
- Males can be affected, causing balanitis xerotica obliterans.
- Women affected between the ages of <5 and 94 years.
- Associated with autoimmune disease such as thyroid disease.
- Oestrogen, testosterone, cryotherapy or laser ablation are not useful therapies.
- Histology – epidermal atrophy with loss of rete ridges, dermal oedema with hyalinization of collagen and subdermal chronic inflammatory infiltrate.

## 3.58 Answers

A **True** – Affects mucous membranes (including mouth) and cutaneous surfaces such as inner surfaces of wrists and legs.
B **True** – Vagina involved causing scarring with stenosis/adhesions.
C **False** – Mild vulval symptoma can be treated with topical corticosteroids.
D **True** – Severe symptoms require systemic steroids or azathioprine.

Note:
- Vulval lesions present as white patterned areas which may be elevated and thickened.

### 3.59 Answers

**A** **True** – Paget's disease is associated with adenocarcinoma of the apocrine sweat gland, other genital tract (vulva, cervix, endometrium, ovary) and urinary tract malignancies.

**B** **False** – Vulval lichen sclerosis should be treated with topical corticosteroids.

**C** **True** – Pruritus is a recognized feature of VIN.

**D** **False** – 95% of vulval carcinomas are squamous cell carcinomas, ~5% are melanomas. Adenocarcinomas of Bartholin's gland, basal cell carcinoma and verrucous carcinoma are rare.

### 3.60 Answers

**A** **False.**

**B** **False.**

**C** **True** – Behçet disease is a rare disorder of recurrent oral and genital ulceration, eye lesions and multiple skin lesions.

**D** **True.**

Note:
- Criteria to establish diagnosis of Behçet disease:
  1. Mucocutaneous lesions (oral ulcers – recurrent, at least three times per year).
  2. Patients must also meet two of the following four criteria: recurrent genital ulcerations, eye lesions (uveitis or retinal vasculitis), positive pathergy test (trauma-induced lesions), skin lesions.
- Recurrence and relapse are common.
- Multiple organs involved including eyes, mouth, lungs, joints, CNS, GI tract and genitalia.
- Granulomas present on histological examination.

### 3.61 Answers

**A** **True** – Perianal Crohn's disease may involve the vulva.

**B** **False.**

**C** **False.**

**D** **False.**

### 3.62 Answers

**A** **False** – Cystic.

**B** **False** – Found on the cervix.

**C** **False** – Rare but cystic.

**D** **False** – Cystic typically, although solid tumours reported.

## 3.63 Answers

**A** True.
**B** False.
**C** True.
**D** False – Call-Exner bodies found in granulosa cell tumours of the ovary.

Note:

- Adenocarcinoma in-situ is similar to Paget's disease of the breast.
- Associated with pruritus and appears as a red crusted plaque with sharp edges.
- Confirm diagnosis by biopsy.
- Associated with adenocarcinoma of the apocrine sweat gland, other genital tract (vulva, cervix, endometrium, ovary), urinary tract and GI malignancies such as rectal adenocarcinoma.
- Treated by vulvectomy.

## 3.64 Answers

**A** True – Presents with pruritus vulvae although 20–45% of cases are asymptomatic.
**B** True – More common in immunocompromised.
**C** True – Spontaneous regression may occur. Therefore, expectant management in asymptomatic young women as they can be followed-up with repeated biopsies if there are suspicious changes.
**D** True – $CO_2$ laser vaporization may be effective although the depth of destruction for adequate treatment is unknown.

Note:

- Uncertain natural history, multifocal nature of disease and mutilating potential of surgery make treatment difficult. Malignant change more likely in older women, immunocompromised and those with other genital tract malignancies.

## 3.65 Answers

**A** False.
**B** False.
**C** False.
**D** False.

Note:

- Risk factors for vulval cancer: age – majority of patients are over the age of 60 years; lichen sclerosus; HPV, especially in younger women; HIV infection; smoking, especially in association with HPV infection; low socioeconomic status; other genital tract cancers, especially cervical cancer.

### 3.66   Answers

**A  False** – 95% of primary tumours are squamous cell carcinomas, and 5% melanomas, basal cell carcinomas, carcinoma of Bartholin's gland and verrucous carcinoma.

**B  True** – Spread to the inguinal and femoral nodes and then the external iliac nodes.

**C  True** – Stage Ia: confined to the vulva or perineum, <2 cm max. diameter, groin nodes not palpable, <1 mm invasion.

**D  True** – Stage Ib: as for Ia but >1 mm invasion.

### 3.67   Answers

**A  True** – Stage III – adjacent spread to lower urethra ± vagina ± anus; unilateral regional lymph node metastases. 20–30% 5-year survival.

**B  True.**

**C  True** – Stage IVa – invasion of upper urethra or bladder mucosa or rectal mucosa or pelvic bone; ± bilateral regional lymph node metastasis; stage IVb – any distant metastasis. 18% 5-year survival.

**D  True.**

Note: Complications of surgical treatment of vulval cancer:

- Stage I – confined to vulva or perineum. Ia <2 cm diameter and <1 mm invasion; Ib <2 cm diameter, >1 mm invasion, no groin nodes palpable. 76% 5-year survival.
- Stage II – confined to vulva or perineum, >2 cm diameter.

### 3.68   Answers

**A  True** – Wound breakdown and infection - less common/severe with triple incision.

**B  True.**

**C  True** – Chronic leg oedema.

**D  True.**

Note:

- Complications of surgical treatment of vulval cancer: wound breakdown and infection, VTE, osteitis pubis, secondary haemorrhage, chronic leg oedema and lymphocysts, numbness and paraesthesia over anterior thigh, loss of body image and impaired sexual function.

### 3.69   Answers

**A  False** – 92% of primary tumours are squamous cell carcinomas. Other types include malignant melanomas, clear cell adenocarcinomas, endodermal sinus tumours.

**B  True** – Stage I: invasive tumour confined to the vaginal mucosa.

**C  True** – Stage III: involvement of the pelvic side-wall.

**D  False** – Stage II: sub-vaginal infiltration not involving the pelvic side-wall.

Note:

- Stage IV: involvement of bladder/rectal mucosa or spread beyond the pelvis.

**A** **False** – Age-related incidence of clear cell adenocarcinoma of the vagina shows two peaks at 26 and 71 years.

**B** **True** – In utero exposure to DES is associated with an increased risk of clear cell adenocarcinoma of the vagina with a risk of 1:1000 by the age of 34 years. The critical period of exposure is before 18 weeks' gestation.

**C** **False** – Treatment should be by radical surgery ± radiotherapy for invasive lesions.

**D** **False.**

Note:
- Most tumours are situated in the upper vagina.
- 5-year survival rates are similar to those for cervical cancer.

**3.71** **Answers**

**A** **False.**

**B** **False.**

**C** **True** – Most common presenting symptom – peri- or post-menopausal bleeding (50% of patients), followed by amber-coloured vaginal discharge. The syndrome of 'hydrops tubae profluens' in which a patient presents with pelvic mass, profuse watery vaginal discharge, and pelvic pain that is greatly relieved by the sudden disappearance of the mass, is rarely seen but is almost pathognomonic.

**D** **True** – Peak incidence is in the 60–64 years age group.

**3.72** **Answers**

**A** **False.**

**B** **False.**

**C** **False** – See 3.71 C.

**D** **True** – CA-125 may be elevated.

Note:
- ~80% are secondaries, most commonly from ovary, endometrium and gastrointestinal tract. Incidence of primary adenocarcinoma of fallopian tube is 0.3–0.5%.

# 4. Family planning and pelvic infection: Questions

**4.1**  The following are absolute contraindications to the use of the combined oral contraceptive pill:

A  Migraine with aura.
B  Strong family history of breast cancer.
C  Severe inflammatory bowel disease.
D  Personal history of DVT.

**4.2**  The combined oral contraceptive pill:

A  Should be started 3 weeks after delivery at term in a woman who is not breastfeeding.
B  Should be started immediately after a first trimester termination of pregnancy.
C  If started on the first or second day of the cycle, additional contraceptive measures are not required.
D  Is associated with a delay in return of normal fertility after it is discontinued.

**4.3**  Third-generation combined oral contraceptive pills:

A  Contain conjugated equine oestrogen.
B  Contain gestodene.
C  Contain desogestrel.
D  Contain norgestimate.

**4.4**  Third-generation combined oral contraceptive pills:

A  Are associated with an increased risk of venous thromboembolism.
B  Are the preparation of choice in overweight women.
C  Are associated with a lower risk of systemic side effects.
D  Contain levonorgestrel as the progestogen.

**4.5** Use of the combined oral contraceptive pill confers the following benefits:

A Reduction in the incidence of uterine fibroids.
B Reduction in the risk of breast cancer.
C 40% reduction in the risk of ovarian cancer compared to never users.
D 50% reduction in the risk of benign breast disease.

**4.6** The following drugs reduce the efficacy of the combined oral contraceptive pill:

A Phenytoin.
B Sodium valproate.
C Nonoxynol-9.
D Oral ampicillin.

**4.7** The following are indications for discontinuing the combined oral contraceptive pill:

A Hypertension.
B Development of focal migraine.
C Diagnosis of breast cancer in a first-degree relation.
D Jaundice.

**4.8** The following drugs are active when given orally:

A Levonorgestrel.
B Progesterone.
C Desogestrel.
D Ethinyl-oestradiol.

**4.9** The progesterone-only oral contraceptive pill:

A Is associated with an increased risk of ectopic pregnancy when compared to sexually active non-contraceptive users.
B Is associated with an increased risk of ovarian theca-leutein cysts.
C Has a 12-hour window for efficacy.
D In dedicated users has a Pearl index of 0.1/100 woman years.

**4.10** The following progestogens are used in formulations of the progesterone-only pill:

A Medroxyprogesterone acetate.
B Levonorgestrel.
C Norethisterone.
D Ethynodiol diacetate.

**4.11** The progesterone-only contraceptive pill:

A Is associated with an increased risk of ovarian follicular cysts.
B Efficacy is reduced by hepatic enzyme-inducing drugs.
C Has suppression of ovulation as its main mode of action.
D Is associated with a delay in return to normal fertility after discontinuation.

**4.12** With respect to the progesterone-only pill:

A Additional precautions are required for 14 days after starting treatment on the first day of menstruation.
B The development of amenorrhoea in the absence of pregnancy indicates anovulation.
C Use confers some protection from sexually transmitted diseases.
D Inhibition of ovulation occurs in over 90% of women.

**4.13** The progesterone-only pill is associated with:

A Poor cycle control.
B Intrahepatic cholestasis.
C Fibroadenosis of the breast.
D Inhibition of lactation.

**4.14** The progesterone-only pill is associated with:

A Endometrial decidualization.
B An increased incidence of functional ovarian cysts.
C Endometrial pseudo-decidualization.
D No delay in return to normal fertility after treatment is stopped.

**4.15** Non-contraceptive benefits of depot medroxyprogesterone acetate include:

A Reduction in the risk of pelvic inflammatory disease.
B Reduction in the risk of endometrial cancer.
C Reduced risk of endometriosis.
D Reduced risk of ectopic pregnancy compared to sexually active non-contraceptive users.

**4.16** The etonorgestrel-releasing implant:

A Has a Pearl index of 2.0.
B Reliably inhibits ovulation.
C Is associated with an immediate return of fertility on removal.
D Inhibits the LH surge thereby preventing ovulation.

**4.17** Mifepristone:

A Is a 19-ketosteroid and a progesterone antagonist.
B Is a 19-norsteroid and a progesterone antagonist.
C Is used as a medical alternative to surgical pregnancy termination at 10 weeks' gestation.
D Can be used with diclofenac as analgesia.

**4.18** Mifepristone:

A Can safely be used in patients with renal failure.
B Is contraindicated in smokers over the age of 35 years.
C Results in decreased myometrial sensitivity to prostaglandins.
D Blocks myometrial oestrogen receptors.

**4.19** The following are recognized complications/side effects of mifepristone administration:

A Nausea and vomiting.
B Rash.
C Headache.
D Hypertension.

**4.20** The following are recognized complications of misoprostol used in early medical termination of pregnancy:

A Pyrexia of 38°C.
B Diarrhoea.
C Nausea and vomiting.
D Acute exacerbation of asthma.

**4.21** With respect to post-coital contraception:

A Hormonal post-coital contraception should not be administered if >72 h have elapsed after unprotected intercourse.

B Oestrogen-only regimens are less effective at preventing pregnancy than oestrogen + progestogen regimens.

C The progesterone-only (Ho and Kwan) regimen is more effective than the oestrogen + progesterone (Yuzpe) regimen.

D The Ho and Kwan regimen uses levonorgestrel 500 μg × 2 doses 12 h apart.

**4.22** The following agents are effective post-coital contraceptives:

A Mifepristone.

B Misoprostol.

C Ethinyl-oestradiol.

D Levonorgestrel.

**4.23** With respect to post-coital contraception:

A The Yuzpe regimen uses 100 μg ethinyloestradiol + 0.5 mg levonorgestrel × 2 doses 12 h apart.

B The Yuzpe regimen is associated with fewer side effects compared to the Ho and Kwan regimen.

C The intrauterine contraceptive device may be fitted up to 5 days after unprotected intercourse.

D The intrauterine contraceptive device may be fitted up to 5 days after the most probable calculated date of ovulation.

**4.24** The following drugs reduce the efficacy of the levonorgestrel-only post-coital contraceptive:

A Phenytoin.

B Ampicillin.

C Sodium valproate.

D Carbamazepine.

**4.25** The levonorgestrel-releasing intrauterine system (MIRENA):

A Is associated with a lower risk of ectopic pregnancy compared to sexually active non-contraceptive users.

B Is associated with a lower risk of functional ovarian cysts compared to copper IUDs.

C Is licensed for the treatment of menorrhagia in the UK.

D Is licensed as an intrauterine contraceptive device for 5 years.

4.26 The levonorgestrel-releasing intrauterine system (MIRENA):

A Is associated with an increased risk of amenorrhoea compared to copper IUDs.

B Is associated with a significant increase in menstrual blood loss.

C Contains 500 mg levonorgestrel.

D Releases levonorgestrel at the rate of 30 µg per day.

4.27 The following are absolute contraindications to IUCD fitting:

A Three previous caesarean sections.

B Major distortion of the uterine cavity.

C Active pelvic inflammatory disease.

D A past history of ectopic pregnancy.

4.28 With respect to IUCDs:

A The GyneFix IUCD is licensed for 8 years.

B The Cu T 380 is licensed for 8 years.

C The Multiload Cu 375 is licensed for 5 years.

D A device fitted after the age of 40 years can safely be left in situ until 1 year after the menopause.

4.29 With respect to IUCDs:

A There is a six-fold increase in the risk of PID in the first 20 days following insertion.

B The risk of PID increases significantly with increasing duration of use.

C The risk of uterine perforation is 1 in 200 insertions.

D The GyneFix IUCD is unsuitable for nulliparous women.

4.30 With respect to IUCDs:

A The GyneFix IUCD is associated with a significantly lower expulsion rate compared to the Cu T 380.

B If an intrauterine pregnancy occurs, removal of the IUCD is associated with a 50% increase in the risk of spontaneous miscarriage.

C The MIRENA IUS is associated with a significantly lower pregnancy rate compared to the Cu T 380.

D The efficacy of copper coils is related to the surface area of copper available.

**4.31** The intrauterine contraceptive device:

A Has a 30% expulsion rate during the first 3 months.
B Is associated with an increased risk of endometriosis.
C Is contraindicated in women aged over 40 years.
D Is contraindicated in women with a previous cone biopsy.

**4.32** The PERSONA contraceptive device:

A Measures urinary levels of LH and FSH.
B Needs to be programmed for 1 month before it can be relied upon.
C Is unsuitable for women with a cycle length >35 days.
D Is unsuitable for women with a cycle length <22 days.

**4.33** The PERSONA contraceptive device:

A Can be used effectively by women with polycystic ovary syndrome.
B Needs to be re-programmed after use of emergency contraception.
C Can be used effectively by breastfeeding mothers.
D Measures urinary concentrations of LH and oestron-3-glucouronide.

**4.34** With regard to female sterilization in the UK:

A There is an increased risk of failure if it is performed at the same time as termination of pregnancy.
B The consent of the woman's partner is mandatory.
C Most deaths are due to anaesthetic complications.
D The procedure should not be performed during menstruation.

**4.35** With regard to female sterilization in the UK:

A Failure is the commonest cause of litigation in gynaecological practice.
B It may be performed in an emergency without the woman's consent.
C If performed during the luteal phase, uterine curettage reduces the chance of pregnancy.
D When clips are used, failure more than a year later is typically the result of clip misapplication.

**4.36** With respect to tubal ligation:

A The risk of ectopic pregnancy is lower in sterilized women compared to non-sterilized fertile women.
B The 10-year cumulative life-table probability of failure of sterilization is 0.5%.
C The risk of laparotomy associated with laparoscopic sterilization is 1:10 000.
D The risk of death associated with laparoscopy is 1:12 000.

**4.37** With respect to tubal ligation:

A Tubal ligation has been shown to be associated with an increased risk of menorrhagia in women below the age of 30 years.
B Use of diathermy for tubal occlusion is associated with an increased risk of ectopic pregnancy.
C Diathermy bowel injury typically presents within 48 hours of surgery.
D Mini-laparotomy is associated with a significantly greater risk of major morbidity compared to laparoscopy.

**4.38** With respect to tubal ligation:

A Culdoscopy is an acceptable alternative to laparoscopy.
B Culdoscopy is associated with a lower risk of major morbidity compared to laparoscopy.
C Culdoscopy is associated with a higher rate of technical difficulty than laparoscopy.
D The Pomeroy technique uses non-absorbable suture to tie the base of a loop of fallopian tube.

**4.39** With respect to tubal ligation:

A Filshie clips should be applied at right angles to the ampulla of the fallopian tube.
B Filshie clip should be applied 4–5 cm from the cornu.
C Topical application of local anaesthesia to the fallopian tubes significantly reduces post-op pain scores.
D If diathermy is required, monopolar diathermy is preferred to bipolar diathermy.

4.40  Vasectomy is associated with:

A  A fall in plasma testosterone concentrations in the first 6 months.
B  A failure rate of 1:2000.
C  The development of antisperm antibodies in over 40% of patients.
D  Epididimo-orchitis as an immediate postoperative complication.

4.41  Vasectomy:

A  Is associated with an increased risk of coronary artery disease.
B  Is associated with epididymo-orchitis, which typically occurs in the first year post-op.
C  Is associated with a reduction in risk of prostate cancer.
D  Is associated with an increased risk of autoimmune disease.

4.42  With respect to vaginal discharge:

A  10% of women have recurrent vaginal discharge.
B  The normal vaginal pH is 3.8–4.4.
C  The prevalence of *Trichomonas vaginalis* in STD clinics is <1%.
D  Use of the COCP predisposes to recurrent vaginal candidiasis.

4.43  Bacterial vaginosis:

A  Is characterized by a lowered vaginal pH.
B  Typically presents with a grey offensive frothy vaginal discharge.
C  Is characterized by the presence of Gram-positive coccobacilli in vaginal discharge.
D  Clue cells are vaginal epithelial cells covered by adherent bacteria which obscure the cellular outline and nucleus.

4.44  *Trichomonas vaginalis*:

A  Is a flagellated protozoa.
B  Strawberry cervix is a classical manifestation.
C  Is associated with increased vaginal pH.
D  Is sensitive to metronidazole.

4.45   The following are risk factors for vaginal candidiasis:

A  Pregnancy.
B  Use of COCP.
C  Use of broad-spectrum antibiotics.
D  Immunosuppression.

4.46   *Actinomyces israelii*:

A  Spreads via lymphatics.
B  If identified on cervical smear is a contraindication to subsequent use of IUDs.
C  Is associated with sinus formation.
D  Is a Gram-positive aerobic organism.

4.47   *Actinomyces israelii*:

A  May be diagnosed on routine cervical smear.
B  Is sensitive to penicillin.
C  Is sensitive to tetracycline.
D  Is associated with sulphur granules in pus.

4.48   *Chlamydia trachomatis*:

A  Is a Gram-negative intracellular organism.
B  Cannot be cultured in the laboratory.
C  Produces intracellular particles called reticulate bodies which are infectious.
D  Produces infectious particles known as elementary bodies.

4.49   *Chlamydia trachomatis*:

A  Is sensitive to erythromycin.
B  Is sensitive to clindamycin.
C  Is typically resistant to azythromycin.
D  Is associated with silent relatively asymptomatic PID.

4.50   Condylomata accuminata:

A  Are most commonly found at the fourchette.
B  Typically regress during pregnancy.
C  Typically appear within 5–7 days of infection.
D  Do not obstruct labour.

**4.51** Condylomata accuminata:

A Are caused by *Treponema pallidum* infection.
B Are characteristically associated with inguinal lymphadenopathy.
C May be treated with topical 5-flurouracil.
D Should not be treated with cryotherapy.

**4.52** The erythrocyte sedimentation rate:

A Is the rate of fall of red cells in a column of blood.
B Is a measure of the acute phase response.
C When raised, reflects an increase in plasma concentration of large proteins.
D Increases with age.

**4.53** The following organisms are typically associated with acute PID:

A *Neisseria gonorrhoea.*
B *Chlamydia trachomatis.*
C *Actinomyces israelii.*
D *Trichomonas vaginalis.*

**4.54** The following are essential for a clinical diagnosis of acute PID:

A Cervical excitation.
B Adnexal tenderness.
C Offensive vaginal discharge.
D A history of unprotected sexual intercourse.

# Answers

### 4.1 Answers

**A** True.
**B** False.
**C** True.
**D** True.

Note: WHO group 4 (conditions for which COCP use is associated with unacceptable health risks):

- Previous thrombosis, ischaemic heart disease.
- Cardiomyopathies, active Kawasaki disease.
- BMI > 39, BP > 160/100.
- Severe diabetes mellitus, focal migraine.
- Thrombophilia, 4 weeks before major surgery – 2 weeks after full mobility.
- Active liver disease, severe inflammatory bowel disease.
- Undiagnosed genital tract bleeding/pregnancy.
- Acute porphyria/SLE, uncorrected valvular heart disease.
- TIAs/cerebral haemorrhage, altitude >4500 m, trophoblastic disease – until HCG undetectable.
- Hyperprolactinaemia (seek specialist advice).

### 4.2 Answers

**A** True – Start 3 weeks after delivery if woman is not breastfeeding – increased risk of VTE if started earlier. If started after day 21, use additional method of contraception for 7 days.
**B** True – Start on same day as first trimester miscarriage or TOP.
**C** True – Additional contraception is not required if started on day 1–2 of the cycle.
**D** True – There is a delay in ovulation in women who discontinue COCP. Women who stopped a barrier method to achieve a planned pregnancy conceived most quickly: 54% were delivered after 1 year vs 39% of IUCD and 32% of oral contraceptive users.

### 4.3 Answers

**A** False.
**B** True – Third-generation COCP contains: desogestrel, gestodene and norgestimate.
**C** True.
**D** True.

### 4.4 Answers

**A** True – Risk of VTE: healthy women not taking COCP – 5/100 000; second-generation COCP user – 15/100 000; third-generation COCP user (desogestrel or gestodene) – 25/100 000; pregnancy – 60/100 000.
**B** False – These pills should therefore not be used in overweight women.
**C** False.
**D** False.

## 4.5 Answers

**A** True.

**B** False – Increase in the risk of developing breast cancer (relative risk 1.24 in current users).

**C** True – Use for 4 and 8 years associated with a 40% and 51% reduction in risk of ovarian cancer, respectively, and a 54% and 66% reduction in risk of ovarian cancer.

**D** True – Reduction in risk of benign breast disease and uterine fibroids.

## 4.6 Answers

**A** True – Phenytoin (*not* valproate) is a hepatic enzyme-inducing drugs. Others include: carbamazepine, griseofulvin, phenobarbital, primidone, rifampicin (and rifabutin), modafinil. Take additional contraceptive precautions during use and for 7 days after use – start next packet without a break if 7 days runs beyond the end of a packet. For rifampicin/rifambutin – use additional contraception for at least 4 weeks after stopping treatment.

**B** False.

**C** False.

**D** True – Broad-spectrum antibiotics impair bacterial flora responsible for enterohepatic circulation of ethinyl-oestradiol. Additional contraception during treatment and for 7 days after treatment as described in A.

## 4.7 Answers

**A** True – Untreated hypertension is an absolute contraindication to use of COCP.

**B** True –Focal migraine is an absolute contraindication to use of COCP.

**C** False – A family history of breast cancer is not a contraindication to COCP.

**D** True – Active liver disease (jaundice) is an absolute contraindication to use of COCP.

## 4.8 Answers

**A** True.

**B** False – Progesterone is not used therapeutically. Progestogens such as levonorgestrel and desogestrel and oestrogens such as ethinyl-oestradiol are active on oral administration

**C** True.

**D** True.

### 4.9 Answers

**A False** – Associated with increased risk of ovarian follicular cysts and of ectopic pregnancy compared to COCP, but decreased risk compared to sexually active non-contraceptive user.

**B False.**

**C False** – One tablet daily taken from day 1 of the cycle and taken continuously. Should be taken at the same time every day and within 3 hours at the most.

**D False** – Pearl index is 1.2/100 woman year.

### 4.10 Answers

**A False.**

**B True** – Levonorgestrel 30 μg.

**C True** – Norethisterone 350 μg.

**D True** – Ethynodiol diacetate 500 μg.

Note:
- Norgestrel 75 μg.

### 4.11 Answers

**A True** – See 4.9A.

**B True** – See 4.6A.

**C False** – Suppresses ovulation in ~40%. This is unpredictable and varies between cycles resulting in irregular menstruation. Its main effect is on cervical mucus.

**D False** – Prompt return to normal fertility on stopping treatment.

### 4.12 Answers

**A False** – One tablet daily taken from day 1 of the cycle and taken continuously. Additional precautions not required when starting treatment.

**B True** – 10–15% of women have complete inhibition of ovarian activity and are amenorrhoeic. ~50% have regular ovulatory cycles with a normal luteal phase and a normal menstrual cycle. 35–40% have inconsistent suppression of ovarian activity and poor cycle control.

**C True** – Effect on cervical mucus may confer some protection against pelvic infection.

**D False** – See A.

### 4.13 Answers

**A True** – See 4.12A.

**B False** – Intrahepatic cholestasis is thought to be related to oestrogen.

**C False.**

**D False** – Does not affect lactation.

## 4.14 Answers

**A** **False** – Not associated with endometrial decidualization. Associated with endometrial atrophy.
**B** **True** – Associated with increased incidence of ovarian follicular cysts.
**C** **False.**
**D** **True** – Prompt return to normal fertility after treatment is stopped.

## 4.15 Answers

**A** **True** – Reduced risk of PID, endometriosis and fibroids.
**B** **True** – Decreased risk of endometrial cancer comparable to COCP.
**C** **True.**
**D** **True** – Decreased risk of ectopic pregnancy compared to sexually active non-contraceptive users. Risk of ectopic pregnancy is increased compared to COCP.

Note:
• Reduced menstrual blood loss and anaemia.

## 4.16 Answers

**A** **False** – Pearl index 0–1/100 woman-years.
**B** **True** – Acts by ovarian suppression, endometrial effects, cervical mucus thickening.
**C** **True** – Rapid return of fertility – 90% of women ovulate within 30 days of stopping treatment.
**D** **True.**

Note:
• Lasts 3 years but efficacy may be lower during the third year in overweight women.

## 4.17 Answers

**A** **False.**
**B** **True** – Derivative of norethindrone (19-norsteroid) – similar chemical structure to progesterone/glucocorticoids.
**C** **False** – Licensed for use in early medical termination of pregnancy up to 63 days from LMP.
**D** **False** – Avoid aspirin/NSAIDs for at least 8–12 days after mifepristone.

## 4.18 Answers

**A** **False.**
**B** **True.**
**C** **False** – Increases the sensitivity of the myometrium to prostaglandins and blocks progesterone receptors.
**D** **False.**

Note: Contraindications to mifepristone:
• Suspected ectopic pregnancy, chronic adrenal insufficiency, long-term corticosteroid therapy, haemorrhagic disorders, anticoagulant therapy, smokers over the age of 35.

### 4.19 Answers

A True.
B True.
C True.
D False.

Note:
- Recognized side effects/complications of mifepristone: vaginal bleeding, malaise, headache, nausea, vomiting, rash.

### 4.20 Answers

A **False** – Pyrexia is typically low grade.
B True.
C True.
D **False** – Unlike carboprost and dinoprostone, misoprostol is not associated with bronchospasm.

### 4.21 Answers

A **False** – Hormonal methods may be used after 72 h but are associated with greater failure.
B **False** – Oestrogen-only regimens appear to be more effective but are associated with more side effects and are no longer used.
C **True** – Ho and Kwan regimen is more effective than the Yuzpe regimen in preventing pregnancy.
D **False** – 750 µg levonorgestrel 12 h apart x2 doses.

### 4.22 Answers

A True.
B False.
C True.
D True.

Note:
- Suitable agents for post-coital contraception: oestrogen, oestrogen + progestogen, progestogen only, danazol, mifepristone, IUCD.

### 4.23 Answers

A **True** – Yuzpe regimen: 100 µg ethinyl-oestradiol + 500 µg levonorgestrel 12 h apart given within 72 h of unprotected intercourse.
B **False** – Ho and Kwan regimen (750 µg levonorgestrel x2 doses 12 h apart is associated with significantly fewer side effects.
C **True** – Copper IUCD can be fitted up to 5 days after unprotected intercourse or after the most probable day of ovulation.
D True.

## 4.24 Answers

A **True** – Effectiveness is reduced by hepatic enzyme-inducing drugs such as phenytoin, carbamazepine, rifampicin – increase dose to 2.25 mg single dose.

B **False** – Efficacy is not affected by broad-spectrum antibiotics.

C **False.**

D **True.**

## 4.25 Answers

A **True** – Low rate of ectopic pregnancy (0.02/100 woman years compared to 0.25/100 woman-years for the Nova T and 1.2–1.6/100 woman-years for sexually active women not using contraception).

B **False** – Increased incidence of functional ovarian cysts compared to copper IUD users.

C **True** – Licensed for contraception for 5 years and for the treatment of menorrhagia.

D **True.**

## 4.26 Answers

A **True** – 35% amenorrhoea rate at 1 year.

B **False.**

C **False** – Contains 52 mg levonorgestrel.

D **False** – Levonorgestrel released at the rate of 20 μg/day.

Note:

- In the management of menorrhagia, reduction in menstrual blood loss of up to 97% after 12 months of use with an increase in serum ferritin and Hb concentrations.

## 4.27 Answers

A **False.**

B **True.**

C **True.**

D **False.**

Note: IUCD absolute contraindications (WHO 4):

- Current or recent sexually transmitted infection or PID, including post-partum and post-TOP endometritis.
- Distorted uterine cavity.
- Possible pregnancy/undiagnosed vaginal bleeding.
- Pelvic tuberculosis.
- Cervical or endometrial cancer awaiting treatment.
- Malignant gestational trophoblastic disease.

## 4.28 Answers

A **False** – Licensed for 5 years.

B **True**.

C **True**.

D **True** – The Faculty of Family Planning recommends that IUCDs fitted after the 40th birthday need not be changed, since fertility declines rapidly at this age, and should be removed 1 year after the menopause.

## 4.29 Answers

A **True** – Six-fold increase in risk of developing PID in the first 20 days following insertion compared with any other time. Thereafter the risk of infection remains constant at 1.4/1000 women.

B **False**.

C **False** – Risk of perforation = 1.2/1000 insertions.

D **False** – The GyneFix IUCD is not specifically contraindicated in nullips.

## 4.30 Answers

A **True** – GyneFix has a significantly lower expulsion rate (3.0/100 women at 3 years) compared to Cu T 380 (7.38/100 women at 3 years).

B **False** – If pregnancy occurs, removal of IUCD reduces the risk of miscarriage.

C **False** – MIRENA has similar efficacy to Cu T 380.

D **True** – The efficacy of Cu IUCDs is related to the surface area of Cu and devices containing 200–250 mm² of Cu are no longer suitable for long-term contraception.

## 4.31 Answers

A **False** – Expulsion risk is highest in the first year and especially if the IUCD is inserted immediately postpartum (up to 10%).

B **False** – Not associated with endometriosis.

C **False**.

D **False**.

Note: Contraindications to IUCDs:

- Relative (WHO 3): immunosuppression including HIV/AIDS, high risk of sexually transmitted disease, menorrhagia (except IUS), benign trophoblastic disease, up to 4 weeks post-partum (risk of perforation/expulsion), ovarian cancer awaiting treatment.
- Absolute (WHO 4): current or recent sexually transmitted infection or PID, including post-partum and post-TOP endometritis, distorted uterine cavity, possible pregnancy/undiagnosed vaginal bleeding, pelvic tuberculosis, cervical or endometrial cancer awaiting treatment, malignant gestational trophoblastic disease.

## 4.32 Answers

**A** **False** – Measures levels of LH and oestron-3-glucouronide in early morning urine.

**B** **False** – Needs to be programmed for 3 months (test urine for 16 days in the first month and 8 days in subsequent months) before device can be relied upon.

**C** **True** – Not suitable for the following groups of women: cycle length <23 days or >35 days, PCOS, breastfeeding, menopausal symptoms, women taking hormonal medication.

**D** **True.**

## 4.33 Answers

**A** **False** – See 4.32C.

**B** **True.**

**C** **False** – See 4.32C.

**D** **True** – See 4.32A.

## 4.34 Answers

**A** **True** – Post-partum or post-TOP tubal ligation is associated with increased regret rate and possibly increased failure rate.

**B** **False** – Although not a legal requirement, it is good practice to involve both partners in the decision making.

**C** **False** – 39% of deaths from female sterilization are related to complications of anaesthesia.

**D** **False** – Can be performed at any time but should be avoided during the luteal phase in a sexually active woman not using contraception.

## 4.35 Answers

**A** **True** – Failure is commonest cause of litigation in gynaecology (~19% of cases).

**B** **False** – Should never be performed without consent; it is not a life-saving procedure.

**C** **False** – Uterine curettage in these circumstances would be an illegal termination of pregnancy.

**D** **False** – Late failure is usually due to re-canalization.

## 4.36 Answers

**A** **True** – Risk of ectopic pregnancy is 4–76% depending on method of sterilization. Risk of ectopic pregnancy is however lower in sterilized than non-sterilized fertile women.

**B** **False** – 10-year cumulative life table probability of failure = 16.6 per 1000 for female sterilization.

**C** **False** – Risk of unintended laparotomy at sterilization is 1.4–3.1/1000.

**D** **True** – Risk of death is 1:12 000.

### 4.37 Answers

**A** **False** – Not associated with increased risk of menorrhaghia if performed after the age of 30 years. Limited data on younger women.

**B** **True** – Diathermy should not be used as primary method – less reversible and carries increased risk of ectopic pregnancy.

**C** **False** – Unrecognized diathermy injury to bowel typically presents 3–7 days later with abdominal pain and fever but can present up to 2 weeks post-op.

**D** **False** – When trained staff and equipment are available, laparoscopy is quicker (by 5 min) and carries a lower (minor) morbidity rate compared to mini-laparotomy, with no significant difference in major morbidity rate.

### 4.38 Answers

**A** **False** – Culdoscopy should not be used – associated with unacceptably high incidence of technical difficulty and major complications.

**B** **False.**

**C** **True.**

**D** **False** – Pomeroy technique uses absorbable suture to tie the base of a loop of tube near the mid-portion and cutting off the top of the loop. Destroys 3–4 cm of tube, making reversal more difficult.

### 4.39 Answers

**A** **False** – Filshie clips should be applied at right angles to the isthmic portion of the tube, 1–2 cm from the cornu, making sure the whole width of the tube is encased in the clip.

**B** **False.**

**C** **True** – Topical application of local anaesthesia to the fallopian tubes whenever mechanical occlusive devices are being applied significantly reduces post-op pain scores and post-op requirement of opiates.

**D** **False** – Diathermy should not be used as primary method – less reversible and carries increased risk of ectopic pregnancy. Bipolar diathermy is safer and preferable to monopolar.

### 4.40 Answers

**A** **False.**

**B** **True.**

**C** **True** – Associated with development of antisperm antibodies in ~70% of men. This raised concerns about a possible increase in the risk of autoimmune diseases but this has been shown not to be the case.

**D** **False** – Associated with an increased risk of epididymo-orchitis, which typically occurs in the first year post-op. The risk of other medical conditions is not increased.

## 4.41 Answers

**A False.**

**B True.**

**C False** – Some data have indicated a modest increase in the risk of prostate cancer.

**D False.**

## 4.42 Answers

**A False** – Recurrent vaginal discharge occurs in <1% of women.

**B True** – Normal vaginal pH 3.8–4.4; maintained by the production of lactic acid by the vaginal epithelium and by lactobacilli.

**C True** – Prevalence of trichomoniasis in GUM clinics 22–77/100 000. Prevalence of 0.1% among women requesting cervical smears.

**D False** – Low dose COCP is not a risk factor for vaginal candidiasis.

Note:
- Physiological discharge increases in pregnancy, mid-cycle and in some women after commencing COCP.

## 4.43 Answers

**A False** – Associated with increased vaginal pH to 4.5–7.0.

**B True** – Presents with thin watery/frothy vaginal discharge with fishy odour.

**C False** – Alteration in the vaginal microbial environment with a reduction in *Lactobaccilus* sp and an increase in facultative and anaerobic bacteria: *G. vaginalis/Bacteroides* sp/*Mobiluncus* sp.

**D True** – Presence of clue cells on wet mount of discharge – vaginal epithelial cells covered with Gram-variable bacteria.

Note:
- 50% of cases are asymptomatic.

## 4.44 Answers

**A True.**

**B True** – On examination, there is usually vulvovaginitis with perivulval intertrigo and petechial haemorrhages on the vaginal wall and ectocervix (strawberry cervix).

**C True** – Associated with increased vaginal pH and bacterial vaginosis.

**D True** – Treat with metronidazole. Partners should also be treated.

Note:
- Sexually transmitted but may be carried asymptomatically in the vagina.
- Causes offensive mucopurulent vaginal discharge with dysuria and vulval soreness.
- Diagnosis confirmed on wet mount microscopy of vaginal fluid (only 50–60% sensitive). Culture is gold standard but requires specialized medium. Clinical diagnosis is unreliable especially in mild cases.
- More common in young sexually active women. Detectable in one-third of sexual partners.

## 4.45 Answers

**A** True.
**B** False.
**C** True.
**D** True.

Note: Risk factors for vaginal candidiasis:

- Immunosuppression – HIV, steroids or other immunosuppressive agents.
- Diabetes mellitus.
- Vaginal douching, bubble bath, tight clothing/tights.
- Pregnancy.
- High-dose COCP (not the current low-dose COCP).
- Broad-spectrum antibiotic therapy.

## 4.46 Answers

**A** False.
**B** False.
**C** **True** – Characterized by the presence of sulphur granules in pus, sinus formation and lack of lymphatic involvement.
**D** **False** – Gram-positive branching filamentous bacilli which form pseudo-mycelium. Strictly anaerobic and without acid-fast staining.

Note:

- Associated with use of IUCD.

## 4.47 Answers

**A** **True** – Diagnosis may be made on cervical smear.
**B** **True** – Sensitive to penicillin/tetracyclines.
**C** True.
**D** **True** – See 4.46C.

## 4.48 Answers

**A** True.
**B** **False** – Can only be grown in cell culture systems.
**C** **False** – Intracellular form is known as a reticulate body – non-infectious and does not survive outside the cell; replicates by binary fission to produce intracellular inclusions.
**D** **True** – Infectious particle is known as an elementary body – attaches to susceptible host cells and is taken up by phagocytosis.

Note:

- Commonest sexually transmitted infection in the UK.
- Various serovars: L1, L2 L3 – lymphogranuloma venereum; A,B,C – trachoma; B-K – genital infection/neonatal conjunctivitis/pneumonia.

## 4.49 Answers

**A** **True** – Sensitive to tetracyclines, erythromycin, azythromycin and amoxicillin.
**B** **True.**
**C** **False.**
**D** **True** – Produces a milder form of salpingitis with insidious onset. May remain in the fallopian tubes for several months in untreated patients. (*N. gonorrhoea* persists for a few days only.)

## 4.50 Answers

**A** **True** – In females, condylomata accuminata (genital warts) are typically found at the posterior fourchette and adjacent labia minora. The perineum, perianal region, vagina and cervix may also be involved. In males they are typically located around the coronal sulcus, on the glans and the frenulum, at the meatus and sometimes on the shaft and surrounding skin. The rectum, anal canal and perianal areas can also be involved.
**B** **False.**
**C** **False** – Typically appear 2–8 months after the infection but may take several years.
**D** **False** – Genital warts often spread and enlarge in pregnancy, and may complicate labour by bleeding or obstructing labour.

Note:
- Asymptomatic HPV infection is common.
- The signs and symptoms of genital warts include: small, grey, pink or red swellings in the genital area that grow quickly and may coalesce into a cauliflower shape, causing itching or burning the genitalia, discomfort, pain or bleeding with intercourse.

## 4.51 Answers

**A** **False** – HPV infection.
**B** **False.**
**C** **True** – Treatments include: topical treatment with podophyllin, podofilox, 5-fluorouracil cream or trichloroacetic acid (TCA); podophyllin – should not be used in pregnancy; cryotherapy; electrocautery; laser treatment.
**D** **False.**

## 4.52 Answers

**A** **True.**
**B** **True** – Reflects an increase in the plasma concentration of proteins such as fibrinogen and some immunoglobulins.
**C** **True** – Raised in infective, immunological, malignant, ischaemic and traumatic events.
**D** **True** – Increases with age and is higher in females and in patients with anaemia.

### 4.53 Answers

**A** True.
**B** True.
**C** False.
**D** False.

Note: Polymicrobial infection:

- *Chlamydia trachomatis, Neisseria gonorrhoea.*
- Non-gonococcal, non-chlamydial PID – caused by anaerobes (*Bacteriodes/ Peptostreptococcus*), *G. vaginalis*, coliforms, haemolytic and non-haemolytic streptococci and mycoplasma.

### 4.54 Answers

**A** True.
**B** True.
**C** False.
**D** False.

Note: Criteria for clinical diagnosis of acute PID:

- Abdominal tenderness ± rebound tenderness *plus*
- Cervical excitation *plus*
- Adnexal tenderness *plus* one or more of the following: temperature >38°C (present in one-third of women with PID); Gram stain of endocervix positive for Gram-negative intracellular diplococci; leukocytosis >10 000/ml (present in <50% of women with PID); pelvic abscess/inflammatory complex on pelvic examination/ultrasound scan; purulent material in peritoneal cavity.

# 5. Hypertensive disorders of pregnancy: Questions

**5.1** The following are recognized causes of hypertension diagnosed at 12 weeks' gestation:

A Phaeochromocytoma.
B Cushing's syndrome.
C Molar pregnancy.
D Chronic renal disease.

**5.2** Severe pregnancy-induced hypertension is associated with:

A Reduced renal uric acid clearance.
B Elevated maternal serum cortisol concentration.
C Hypernatraemia.
D Hyperkalaemia.

**5.3** With respect to drug therapy in severe pregnancy-induced hypertension:

A The dose of methyldopa should not exceed 2 g per 24 h.
B Methyldopa does not cross the placenta.
C Nightmares are a recognized complication of methyldopa.
D Coombs' positive haemolytic anaemia is a recognized complication of methyldopa.

**5.4** With respect to drug therapy in severe pregnancy-induced hypertension:

A Headache is a recognized side effect of hydralazine therapy.
B Hydralazine may be used for long-term treatment of hypertension.
C Intravenous labetalol has a faster onset of action than intravenous hydralazine.
D Labetalol is a combined alpha and beta antagonist.

5.5 Pre-eclampsia is associated with:

A Reduced intravascular volume.
B Thrombocytopenia.
C Haemo-concentration.
D Increased renal perfusion.

5.6 The following are side effects of methyldopa:

A Depression.
B Abnormal liver function tests.
C Nightmares.
D Rash.

5.7 The following are indications for delivery in a woman with pre-eclampsia at 30 weeks' gestation:

A Uncontrollable hypertension.
B 24 h urine protein excretion of 3 g.
C Hyperreflexia.
D Development of HELLP syndrome.

5.8 In a woman with severe pre-eclampsia, the following are contraindications to regional anaesthesia:

A Raised liver enzymes.
B Platelet count <80 000/ml.
C Prolonged PT and APTT.
D Uncontrollable hypertension.

5.9 Eclampsia:

A Is more common in the antenatal than in the postnatal period.
B Carries a 5% mortality.
C Is the commonest cause of direct maternal mortality in the UK.
D May occur in the absence of hypertension and proteinuria.

5.10 In the management of a woman who has suffered an eclamptic fit:

A Muscle weakness is a recognized complication of magnesium sulphate therapy.
B Magnesium sulphate is metabolized principally by the liver.
C The maintenance dose of magnesium sulphate should be reduced if liver enzymes are elevated.
D The maintenance dose of magnesium sulphate should be increased if urine output is >100 ml/h.

5.11 The following are recognized complications of magnesium sulphate therapy:

A Tachypnoea.
B Flushing of the skin.
C Hyperreflexia.
D Nausea and vomiting.

5.12 In a woman with severe pre-eclampsia, treatment with hydralazine is associated with:

A Increased heart rate.
B Increased cardiac output.
C Increased peripheral resistance.
D Decreased mean arterial pressure.

5.13 The following are recognized side effects of nifedipine therapy:

A Headache.
B Flushing.
C Bradycardia.
D Tachycardia.

5.14 The following are recognized complications of hydralazine therapy:

A Hypotension.
B Flushing.
C Tachycardia.
D Palpitations.

5.15 The following is appropriate management of a woman with severe pre-eclampsia and a urine output of 10 ml in the last hour 5 hours after caesarean section:

A 500 ml of normal saline i.v. over 2 hours.
B Frusemide i.v.
C 500 ml colloid i.v. over 2 hours.
D Assessment of blood loss and blood transfusion if necessary.

5.16 Pre-eclampsia is associated with an increased risk of:

A Post-partum haemorrhage.
B Antepartum haemorrhage.
C Venous thromboembolism.
D IUGR.

# Answers

### 5.1 Answers

**A** True.
**B** True.
**C** True – Molar pregnancy is associated with early onset severe hypertensive disease.
**D** True.

Note:
- Causes of pre-existing hypertension in pregnancy include essential hypertension, renal disease, Cushing's and Conn's syndrome, phaeochromocytoma and coarctation of the aorta.

### 5.2 Answers

**A** True – Renal function is impaired with reduced creatinine/uric acid clearance but electrolyte imbalance does not occur.
**B** False – While CRH concentrations are increased in pre-eclampsia and to a lesser extent in PIH, maternal serum cortisol is not significantly increased.
**C** False.
**D** False.

### 5.3 Answers

**A** True – Max dose of methyldopa: 3 g/24 h but dose of 500 mg four times daily is generally not exceeded in pregnancy.
**B** False.
**C** True.
**D** True – Causes positive Coombs' test in up to 20% of patients.

### 5.4 Answers

**A** True – Hydralazine is an arteriolar vasodilator that provides pure afterload reduction. The typical compensatory response is a reflex tachycardia: headache, nausea and flushing. The response to an intravenous bolus takes up to 20 minutes to manifest.
**B** False.
**C** True – Onset of action is 5 minutes.
**D** True – Labetolol is a mixed alpha- and beta-blocker, so it also has vasodilatory effects (beta effects predominate by a ratio of 7:1).

Note: See 5.14.

## 5.5 Answers

**A** **True** – Intravascular volume is reduced leading to haemoconcentration and raised haematocrit.

**B** **True** – Thrombocytopenia occurs in ~33% of pre-eclamptics and DIC in 7%.

**C** **True** – See A.

**D** **False** – There is mild to moderate reduction in renal perfusion (20%) and GFR (32%; normal GFR 125 ml/min) in pre-eclampsia.

## 5.6 Answers

**A** True.

**B** True.

**C** True.

**D** True.

Note: Side effects of methyldopa:

- GI – dry mouth, stomatitis, hepatitis and abnormal LFT, jaundice, pancreatitis.
- CVS – bradycardia, exacerbation of angina, postural hypotension, oedema, myocarditis/pericarditis.
- CNS – sedation, headache, nightmares, depression/mild psychosis, parkinsonism, Bell's palsy.
- Blood – haemolytic anaemia, bone marrow suppression.
- GU – decreased libido, failure of ejaculation, gynaecomastia, prolactinaemia, amenorrhoea.
- Immune – hypersensitivity reactions with SLE-like syndrome, drug rash.

## 5.7 Answers

**A** True.

**B** False.

**C** False.

**D** True.

Note: Indications for delivery in pre-eclampsia:

- Term fetus.
- Fetal distress/compromise (IUGR with abnormal Dopplers – gestational age dependent).
- Eclampsia.
- Uncontrollable hypertension.
- Maternal symptoms – severe headache/epigastric pain.
- Rapidly deteriorating haematological/biochemical indices.
- HELLP syndrome.

## 5.8 Answers

**A** False.

**B** **True** – Regional analgesia is contraindicated in women with a coagulopathy (platelet count <80 000/ml or prolonged PT/APTT).

**C** True.

**D** **False** – Uncontrollable hypertension is not a contraindication and regional analgesia may be beneficial.

## 5.9 Answers

**A** **False** – 44% postnatal, 38% antenatal and 18% intrapartum.
**B** **False** – Mortality rate 1.8%.
**C** **False** – Second commonest cause of maternal death; VTE is commonest.
**D** **True** – Eclampsia may be the first presentation of hypertensive disease.

## 5.10 Answers

**A** **True** – See 5.11.
**B** **False** – $MgSO_4$ is excreted by the kidneys and not affected by liver function.
**C** **False.**
**D** **False** – Diuresis may occur after delivery and is not an indication for increasing maintenance dose of $MgSO_4$. Dose should be reduced in oliguria.

## 5.11 Answers

**A** **False.**
**B** **True.**
**C** **False.**
**D** **True.**

Note: Side effects of $MgSO_4$ include:

- GI – nausea, vomiting, thirst.
- CVS – hypotension, arrhythmia.
- CNS – respiratory depression, coma, drowsiness, confusion, loss of tendon reflexes, muscle weakness.
- Skin – flushing.

## 5.12 Answers

**A** **True.**
**B** **True** – Hydralazine is an arteriolar vasodilator and provides pure afterload reduction with reduction in mean arterial pressure. The typical compensatory response is a reflex tachycardia with increased cardiac output.
**C** **False.**
**D** **True** – The response to an intravenous bolus takes up to 20 minutes to manifest. Can cause sudden profound hypotension.

Note:

- Hydralazine is not generally used for long-term treatment of hypertension in pregnancy.

## 5.13 Answers

**A** **True.**
**B** **True.**
**C** **False.**
**D** **True.**

Note: Side effects of nifedipine:

- GI – nausea, constipation/diarrhoea, gum hyperplasia.
- GU – frequency of micturition, impotence, gynaecomastia.
- CVS – tachycardia, palpitations, dizziness, oedema.
- CNS – eye pain, visual disturbance, headache, paraesthesia, tremor.
- Skin – rash, flushing.

## 5.14 Answers

**A** True.
**B** True.
**C** True.
**D** True.

Note: Side effects of hydralazine:

- CVS – tachycardia, palpitations, hypotension, fluid retention, dizziness.
- CNS – headache, paraesthesia.
- GI – GI disturbance, abnormal LFT, jaundice.
- Skin – flushing, rash – rare.
- Immune – SLE-like syndrome.

## 5.15 Answers

**A** False.
**B** False – Use of diuretics only indicated when there are obvious signs of fluid overload/pulmonary oedema.
**C** False.
**D** True – Blood loss after caesarean section may cause/compound oliguria.

Note:

- Pre-eclampsia is associated with decreased intravascular volume and renal perfusion leading to oliguria.
- Owing to increased endothelial permeability, fluid challenge may cause pulmonary oedema and should not be undertaken without invasive monitoring.

## 5.16 Answers

**A** True.
**B** True.
**C** True.
**D** True.

Note: Increased risks associated with pre-eclampsia:

- Maternal risks: multisystem organ failure – liver, kidneys, lungs, heart, coagulopathy and brain (eclampsia/haemorrhage); increased risk of PPH/placental abruption; increased risk of VTE and need for operative delivery.
- Fetal risks: impaired placental perfusion is thought to cause the high incidence of fetal loss, IUGR and perinatal mortality. Increased risk of abruption.

# 6. Labour and delivery: Questions

**6.1**  With regard to oblique lie of the fetus:

A The incidence is unaffected by parity.
B Is a recognized indication in labour for classical caesarean section.
C There is a recognized association with fetal renal agenesis.
D The incidence is increased in multiple pregnancy.

**6.2**  With regards to oblique lie of the fetus:

A External cephalic version is recognized management.
B There is a recognized association with fetal neural tube defects.
C In a multiparous woman, elective caesarean section should be performed at 39 weeks' gestation.
D There is a recognized association with placenta previa.

**6.3**  The following statements regarding breech presentation and delivery are true:

A Tentorial tears are a recognized complication of rapid delivery of the head.
B The Mauriceau–Smellie–Veit method is used to deliver the after-coming head.
C There is an increased risk of fetal congenital anomalies.
D External cephalic version should be performed at 36–37 weeks' gestation.

**6.4**  There is an increased risk of face presentation in association with:

A Sternomastoid tumour.
B Contracted maternal pelvis.
C Preterm labour.
D Fetal goitre.

6.5    With regards to face presentation at term:

A  Vaginal delivery may be safely achieved with a mento-anterior position.
B  The incidence is increased by the use of epidural analgesia.
C  The incidence is ~1:150 deliveries.
D  The risk of congenital anomalies is not increased compared to vertex presentations.


6.6    Congenital uterine anomalies in pregnancy are associated with:

A  Recurrent first trimester pregnancy loss.
B  Preterm delivery.
C  Fetal urinary tract anomalies.
D  Breech presentation.


6.7    A 30-year-old primigravida who has been the victim of infibulation is referred to the antenatal clinic at 14 weeks' gestation.

A  A defibulation procedure may be performed in the first stage of labour.
B  A defibulation procedure should not be performed in the second stage of labour.
C  An anterior midline episiotomy may be required during delivery.
D  It is a criminal offence to perform re-infibulation after delivery.


6.8    With regards to the anatomy and mechanism of labour:

A  The sacral promontory is the posterior landmark of the pelvic inlet.
B  The sacro-spinous and sacro-tuberous ligaments form the lateral borders of the pelvic inlet.
C  The transverse diameter of the pelvic inlet is the wider diameter and measures >11 cm.
D  Internal rotation occurs at the bispinous diameter.


6.9    With regards to the anatomy and mechanism of labour:

A  In a well flexed vertex presentation, the occipito-bregmatic diameter presents.
B  In a brow presentation at term, the presenting diameter measures 11 cm.
C  In a breech presentation, the bisacromial diameter presents.
D  The antero-posterior diameter of the pelvic outlet is the wider diameter.

6.10  Induction of labour is associated with:

A  Maternal hyponatraemia.
B  Placental abruption.
C  Uterine rupture.
D  Postpartum haemorrhage.

6.11  Continuous electronic fetal monitoring in labour:

A  Is associated with a lower caesarean section rate.
B  Is recommended if oxytocin is administered.
C  Significantly reduces the risk of fetal acidosis.
D  Should be accompanied by fetal blood sampling if required.

6.12  Late decelerations of the fetal heart rate in labour:

A  Reach their trough at the peak of the contraction.
B  Are secondary to head compression.
C  Are an indication of cord compression.
D  Are always associated with a cord pH < 7.20.

6.13  Fetal acidosis in labour is characteristically associated with:

A  Prolonged uterine hypertonus.
B  Prolonged pregnancy.
C  Fetal intraventricular haemorrhage.
D  Decreased baseline variability on CTG.

6.14  Umbilical cord prolapse is associated with:

A  Increased maternal age.
B  Post-maturity.
C  Breech presentation.
D  Oligohydramnios.

6.15  Rupture of the uterus is associated with:

A  Fetal distress.
B  Haematuria.
C  Blood-stained liquor.
D  Uterine hypertonia.

6.16 Epidural anaesthesia is contraindicated in:

A Pre-eclampsia.
B Breech presentation.
C Preterm labour at 28 weeks' gestation.
D Women within 24 hours of a therapeutic dose of fragmin.

6.17 The following increase the risk of maternal aspiration of gastric contents and the development of Mendelson's syndrome during labour:

A Increased gastric motility.
B Effect of progesterone on the cardiac sphincter.
C Epidural anaesthesia.
D Use of muscle relaxants.

6.18 The following increase the risk of maternal aspiration of gastric contents and the development of Mendelson's syndrome during labour:

A Presence of gastric contents with a high pH.
B The presence of particulate gastric contents.
C The use of cricoid pressure during general anaesthesia.
D Use of pethidine for analgesia.

6.19 The following decrease the risk of maternal aspiration of gastric contents and the development of Mendelson's syndrome during labour:

A Use of oral sodium citrate prior to epidural anaesthesia.
B Use of Gaviscon prior to general anaesthesia for emergency caesarean section.
C Administration of oral metoclopramide and ranitidine prior to caesarean section.
D Administration of i.v. ranitidine prior to emergency caesarean section.

6.20 In amniotic fluid embolism:

A Detection of trophoblast cells in the peripheral circulation is pathognomonic.
B The patient is likely to be a primigravida.
C Over 90% of fatalities occur within 1 hour of the onset of symptoms.
D Maternal mortality occurs in over 80% of reported cases.

**6.21** In amniotic fluid embolism:

A Symptoms characteristically occur before the onset of labour.
B In up to 15% of patients, haemorrhage is the first indication of the condition.
C There is an association with prolonged labour.
D There is an association with the use of oxytocin.

**6.22** Oxytocin:

A Is a polypeptide hormone.
B Is secreted by the anterior pituitary gland.
C Has an antidiuretic effect.
D Should be administered at 2 mU/min to a patient with a prolonged first stage of labour.

**6.23** Oxytocin:

A Causes water intoxication if administered with large volumes of electrolyte-free fluids.
B Should be administered to a woman requesting a physiological third stage of labour.
C Produces tetanic uterine contractions.
D Causes milk ejection.

**6.24** Ergometrine:

A Causes nausea and vomiting.
B Causes hypotension.
C Has a longer duration of action than oxytocin.
D Causes spasmodic uterine contractions.

**6.25** Use of intravenous ergometrine in the third stage of labour is associated with:

A A fall in mean arterial pressure.
B A rise in peripheral resistance.
C Vomiting.
D Palpitations.

6.26 A 34-year-old woman requires operative vaginal delivery for a prolonged second stage of labour:

A The vacuum extractor is significantly more likely to fail compared to the Neville–Barnes forceps.
B There is no significant difference in success rate when the rigid vacuum extractor cup is compared to the sialastic cup.
C Use of the vacuum extractor is associated with a greater need for neonatal phototherapy compared to the forceps.
D Use of the Neville–Barnes forceps is more likely to be associated with maternal worries about the baby.

6.27 The Neville–Barnes forceps:

A Have a pelvic curve.
B Have a cephalic curve.
C Have a sliding lock.
D Can be used to correct asynclitism.

6.28 The Wrigley forceps:

A Have a pelvic curve.
B Have a cephalic curve.
C Have a fixed lock.
D Are most suitable for delivery of the after-coming head during vaginal breech delivery.

6.29 The Kielland forceps:

A Have a pelvic curve.
B Have a cephalic curve.
C Have a sliding lock.
D Can be used to correct for asynclitism.

6.30 Acute inversion of the uterus

A Is a recognized cause of postpartum haemorrhage.
B Is associated with premature delivery.
C Is a recognized consequence of genital prolapse.

**6.31** Acute uterine inversion:

A Occurs more commonly with a fundal placenta.
B Is more common in twin compared to singleton pregnancies.
C Is a consequence of waiting too long for the uterus to contract.
D Should be managed by immediate replacement whether or not the placenta is separated.

**6.32** The following are recognized causes of postpartum collapse in the absence of significant external bleeding:

A Ergometrine administration.
B Eclampsia.
C Uterine rupture.
D Uterine inversion.

**6.33** There is an increased risk of postpartum haemorrhage in association with:

A Multiparity.
B Instrumental delivery.
C Active management of the third stage.
D Haemophilia A carriers.

**6.34** There is an increased incidence of the following conditions in the puerperium compared with pregnancy:

A Thyroiditis.
B Torsion of ovarian cysts.
C Thromboembolism.
D Psychosis.

**6.35** Breastfeeding is contraindicated in:

A Active epilepsy.
B HIV-positive women.
C Inversion of the nipples.
D Prematurity <30 weeks.

**6.36** Breastfeeding is contraindicated in:

A Maternal lithium therapy.
B Maternal warfarin therapy.
C Mastitis.
D Puerperal psychosis.

# Answers

### 6.1 Answers

**A False** – Risk factors for oblique lie include high parity, multiple pregnancy, polyhydramnios, placenta previa, uterine and fetal anomalies (such as neural tube defects, which are also associated with polyhydramnios), pelvic tumours, fibroids.

**B True** – Classical C/S may be indicated although lower segment C/S is usually possible.

**C False** – Fetal renal agenesis is associated with oligohydramnios – this is not a risk factor for oblique or unstable lie.

**D True** – See A.

### 6.2 Answers

**A False** – ECV is not recognized management for oblique or unstable lie.

**B True** – See 6.1A.

**C False** – In a multiparous woman, C/S should be delayed until 40 weeks as spontaneous version may occur. Stabilizing induction is also an option.

**D True** – See 6.1A.

### 6.3 Answers

**A True** – Tentorial tears are a recognized complication of vaginal breech delivery – thought to be due to sudden decompression.

**B True** – After-coming head may be delivered by the Mauriceau–Smellie–Veit or Burns–Marshall manoeuvre or with forceps.

**C True.**

**D False** – ECV should be performed after 37 weeks.

### 6.4 Answers

**A True.**

**B True.**

**C False.**

**D True.**

Note: Risk factors for face presentation include:

- Contracted maternal pelvis or cephalo-pelvic disproportion.
- Multiparity or decreased uterine tone, leading to natural extension of the fetal head.
- Nuchal cord.
- Fetal goitre or sternomastoid tumour – causes extension of fetal neck.
- Anencephaly (>30% of cases of face presentation).
- Other fetal anomalies in up to 60%.

## 6.5 Answers

**A** **True** – Will deliver vaginally only in the mento-anterior position.
**B** **False.**
**C** **False** – Incidence ~1:500 live births.
**D** **False.**

Note:
- 60–80% of face presentations are in mento-anterior position, ~10% are mento-transverse and 20–30% are mento-posterior.
- In the mento-posterior position, the neck is maximally extended and cannot extend further to deliver beneath the symphysis pubis.

## 6.6 Answers

**A** **False** – Uterine anomalies are not associated with recurrent first trimester pregnancy loss.
**B** **True.**
**C** **False** – *Women* with uterine anomalies have an increased risk of urinary tract anomalies and these should be excluded by renal USS or IVP.
**D** **True.**

Note:
- Uterine anomalies are associated with: preterm delivery, malpresentation including breech presentation and unstable lie, increased risk of PPH.

## 6.7 Answers

**A** **True.**
**B** **False.**
**C** **True.**
**D** **True** – If re-infibulation after delivery is requested, it should be made clear that the procedure is illegal in the UK. The consequences of more scarring and subsequent sexual and reproductive difficulties should be explained.

Note:
- Elective defibulation around 20 weeks' gestation reduces lacerations, and avoids lacerations and anterior episiotomy in labour.
- Obstetric complications include: fear of lacerations resulting in requests for C/S; difficulty performing VE in labour; urinary retention and difficulty with catheterization; prolonged labour; need for defibulation in the first stage of labour; anterior or midline episiotomy during delivery; PPH from lacerations; wound infection and retention of lochia causing puerperal sepsis.

## 6.8 Answers

**A True.**

**B False.**

**C True** – The female pelvic inlet is oval in shape with the transverse diameter being wider and should be >11 cm.

**D True.**

Note: Landmarks:

- Pelvic inlet: anterior – symphysis pubis + body of pubic bone; posterior – sacral promontory and 'wing' of sacrum; antero-lateral – superior pubic rami and ileo-pectineal line; female pelvic inlet is oval in shape with the transverse diameter being wider and should be >11 cm.
- Mid-cavity: level of ischial spines; site of rotation of the presenting part.
- Pelvic outlet: anterior – symphysis pubis and body of pubic bone; posterior – fifth sacral vertebra; antero-lateral – inferior pubic rami, sacro-spinous and sacro-tuberous ligaments.

## 6.9 Answers

**A False** – Suboccipito-bregmatic diameter is the presenting diameter in a well flexed vertex presentation with an occipito-anterior position.

**B False** – In brow presentation at term, the presenting diameter is the mento-vertical diameter ~13 cm.

**C False** – The presenting diameter in a breech presentation is the bi-tronchanteric diameter.

**D True** – The pelvic outlet is diamond-shaped with the antero-posterior diameter being wider.

## 6.10 Answers

**A True.**

**B True.**

**C True.**

**D True.**

Note: Complications of induction of labour:

- Failure.
- Uterine hyperstimulation – fetal hypoxia.
- Fetal distress – more common in induced labour.
- Cord prolapse.
- Placental abruption – more likely to occur at membrane rupture.
- Uterine rupture.
- Neonatal hyperbilirubinaemia – associated with use of oxytocin.
- PPH secondary to uterine hypotonia.
- Hyponatraemia – associated with use of high doses of oxytocin + administration of electrolyte-poor solutions.
- Inadvertent preterm delivery.

## 6.11 Answers

**A False** – Associated with a significant increase in C/S rate.

**B True** – Because of the risk of fetal acidosis in high-risk labours, including those in which oxytocin is used, electronic fetal monitoring is recommended.

**C False** – No significant reduction in the risk of fetal acidosis.

**D True** – Early detection of fetal acidosis using FBS may prevent up to 50% of neonatal seizures and the use of FBS allows this to occur without an increase in intervention rates due to false-positive CTG.

Note:

- Electronic fetal monitoring in labour is also associated with a significant reduction in neonatal seizures and a significant reduction in perinatal deaths attributable to hypoxia, although there is no overall significant reduction in perinatal mortality.

## 6.12 Answers

**A False** – Late decelerations reach their trough after the peak of the contraction.

**B False** – Fetal head compression is associated with early decelerations.

**C False** – Cord compression is associated with variable decelerations.

**D False** – Late decelerations are an indication of fetal acidosis although there is a high false-positive rate.

## 6.13 Answers

**A True.**

**B True** – Prolonged pregnancy is associated with an increased risk of C/S for fetal distress/acidosis.

**C False** – IVH is a feature of prematurity.

**D True** – CTG features of fetal acidosis in labour include baseline tachycardia, decreased variability and late decelerations. Specificity of CTG abnormalities is poor.

Note: Causes of acute fetal acidosis:

- Maternal: hypotension/hypovolaemia; hypoxia, e.g. fitting; uterine hypertonus.
- Placental: abruption.
- Fetal: cord prolapse, repeated cord compression during labour/true knot in the cord. Based on animal studies, fetal blood flow must be reduced by at least 50% to cause hypoxia.

### 6.14 Answers

A **False.**

B **False.**

C **True** – Risk factors include breech presentation, high head at onset of labour, multiple pregnancy, high parity, preterm labour, polyhydramnios, obstetric manipulations such as forceps delivery, artificial rupture of membranes.

D **False.**

Note:
- Diagnosis usually made when cord is identified at the introitus or in the vagina on examination.
- Diagnosis is suggested by the sudden appearance of variable decelerations on CTG.
- Manage by prompt C/S unless the cervix is fully dilated with the head below the spines, when delivery by forceps should be undertaken.
- While woman is prepared for delivery, bladder should be filled with 500–700 ml saline to elevate the presenting part and reduce cord compression.
- Other manoeuvres include nursing in knee–chest position face down with the attendant's gloved hand in the vagina to elevate the presenting part.

### 6.15 Answers

A **True** – Signs and symptoms include vaginal bleeding, blood-stained liquor, abdominal pain, fetal parts palpable outside the uterus, fetal distress (abnormal CTG), haematuria, maternal shock.

B **True.**

C **True.**

D **False.**

Note:
- Commonest cause of uterine rupture in developed countries is previous C/S. Other risk factors include previous myomectomy, use of oxytocin/prostaglandins, multiparity, breech version, operative delivery and trauma.
- Contractions do not necessarily cease after rupture.

### 6.16 Answers

A **False.**

B **False.**

C **False.**

D **True** – Regional anaesthesia should be avoided until at least 12 hours after prophylactic dose of LMWH or 24 hours after therapeutic dose. Do not remove epidural catheter until 10–12 hours after dose and do not administer LMWH within 4 hours of removing catheter.

Note:
- Localized or generalized sepsis, coagulopathy (platelet count $<80 \times 10^9$/L or abnormal PT/APTT) and haemorrhage are other contraindications.

## 6.17 Answers

A False.
B True.
C False.
D True.

Note:
- Mendelson's syndrome is characterized by cyanosis and laboured respiration with a pink froth exuding from the respiratory passages.
- Therapeutic strategies to reduce the risk include: fasting of women in labour; measures which may increase gastric pH – use of sodium citrate or oral ranitidine (i.v. if emergency) before anaesthesia for C/S; measures which may reduce the volume of gastric secretions – metoclopramide (pethidine causes gastric stasis and is associated with increased gastric volume); the use of regional rather than general anaesthesia – this virtually eliminates the risk of aspiration provided no sedation is used; pre-oxygenation and the application of cricoid pressure prior to intubation; and protection of the airway by a cuffed endotracheal tube.

## 6.18 Answers

A **False** – Aspiration must occur in the presence of a 'triad' of features:
(1) A stomach that contains gastric secretions at a 'low' pH (<2.5) or one that contains particulate matter; (2) vomiting or regurgitation; (3) depression of the laryngeal reflexes.
B **True.**
C **False** – Pre-oxygenation and the application of cricoid pressure prior to intubation reduces risk of aspiration.
D **True** – Pethidine causes gastric stasis and is associated with increased gastric volume.

## 6.19 Answers

A False.
B False.
C True.
D True.

Note: See 6.17.

## 6.20 Answers

A **False** – Fetal squamous and trophoblast cells are commonly found in the circulation of normal labouring women.
B **False.**
C **False** – 50% die within 1 h of onset of symptoms.
D **True** – Mortality rate ~80–90%.

## 6.21 Answers

**A** False.

**B** True – The first phase of the syndrome is characterized by pulmonary vasospasm, hypoxia and acute respiratory failure. However, coagulopathy with haemorrhage may be the initial presentation in 10–15% of cases.

**C** False.

**D** True.

Note:

- Rare complication – 1:8000–1:30 000 pregnancies.
- Amniotic fluid, fetal cells, hair or other debris enter the maternal circulation, causing cardiorespiratory collapse. Usually a postmortem diagnosis: presence of fetal squames in the maternal pulmonary circulation.
- Risk factors for amniotic fluid embolism: traditionally thought to be multiparous women with a large baby experiencing a short tumultuous labour associated with the use of uterine stimulants; polyhydramnios; uterine rupture; use of oxytocin; intrauterine fetal death; placenta acreta; chorioamnionitis. Typically occurs during labour (may occur during TOP/abdominal trauma). More common with a male fetus. About 40% of patients have a history of allergies.
- There is no association with maternal age.

## 6.22 Answers

**A** True.

**B** False – Produced by the posterior pituitary gland.

**C** True – Similar amino acid sequence to ADH, has antidiuretic effects and may cause water intoxication, especially if high doses are used in association with electrolyte-free fluids.

**D** False – In labour, dose should be titrated to the frequency and strength of contractions with a starting dose of 1–2 mU/min.

## 6.23 Answers

**A** True – See 6.23C.

**B** False – Used in the active management of the third stage.

**C** False – Causes uterine spasms; ergometrine causes titanic contraction.

**D** True – Plays an important role in milk ejection.

## 6.24 Answers

**A** True.

**B** False – Used in the active management of the third stage.

**C** True – Causes uterine spasms; ergometrine causes tetanic contraction.

**D** False.

## 6.25 Answers

**A** False.
**B** True – Associated with nausea and vomiting, headache, dizziness, palpitations, SOB, tinnitus, vasoconstriction causing hypertension, stroke and MI, pulmonary oedema.
**C** True.
**D** True.

Note:
- Ergometrine given i.v./i.m. in combination with oxytocin in active management of the third stage, the combination being more effective than either drug alone. Causes tetanic contraction whereas oxytocin causes uterine spasms.
- Contraindicated in hypertension and cardiac disease.

## 6.26 Answers

**A** True – The use of ventouse compared to forceps is associated with a higher risk of failure, more cephalohaematoma, more retinal haemorrhage. Use of ventouse compared to forceps is associated with less use of regional/general anaesthesia, and less maternal perineal or vaginal trauma.
**B** False – The sialastic ventouse cup is associated with a significant increase in rate of failure compared to the rigid cup but there is a significant reduction in scalp trauma.
**C** False – Ventouse is no more likely to be associated with need for phototherapy.
**D** False – Ventouse is significantly more likely to be associated with maternal worries about the baby.

Note:
- There is no significant difference in C/S rates, low Apgar scores at 5 minutes or long-term follow-up of mothers/babies (5 years) between the methods of operative vaginal delivery.

## 6.27 Answers

**A** True.
**B** True.
**C** False – Have a fixed lock.
**D** False – Used for non-rotational vaginal delivery and should not be used to correct asynclitism.

## 6.28 Answers

**A** True – Non-rotational forceps with pelvic and cephalic curves, and a fixed lock.
**B** True.
**C** True.
**D** False – The after-coming' head in vaginal breech delivery should be delivered with the Piper or Neville–Barnes forceps.

Note:
- Wrigley forceps are used for 'lift-out' vaginal deliveries and for delivery of the head at C/S.

## 6.29 Answers

**A** **False** – Have a cephalic but *no* pelvic curve, and a sliding lock.
**B** **True.**
**C** **True.**
**D** **True** – Offers a single accurate application for correction of asynclitism, rotation and extraction.

Note:
- Kielland forceps are used for rotational operative vaginal delivery.
- The lack of a pelvic curve may increase the risk of vaginal injury during extension of the head at delivery.

## 6.30 Answers

**A** **True** – Presents with abdominal pain, PPH and/or shock in the presence of an inverted (vaginally) or indented (abdominally) uterus.
**B** **False.**
**C** **False.**

Note:
- Uterine inversion occurs in 1:2000 deliveries. Described as complete when the fundus has passed through the cervix.
- Acute inversion occurs in the first 24 hours postpartum. Subacute inversion (24 hours–4 weeks) and chronic inversion (after 4 weeks).

## 6.31 Answers

**A** **True** – See 6.30D.
**B** **False.**
**C** **False.**
**D** **True.**

Note: Management of acute inversion of the uterus:
- Avoid uterotonic agents.
- Resuscitate.
- Leave placenta in situ to prevent haemorrhage and manually replace under anaesthesia, then remove placenta manually (Johnson manoeuvre – replace the last part out first).
- If unsuccessful, replacement following tocolytic administration – $MgSO_4$ or terbutaline under GA.
- Hydrostatic replacement (O'Sullivan's technique) involves manually sealing the introitus as sterile fluid is instilled into the vagina and is effective.

### 6.32 Answers

**A** False.
**B** True.
**C** True.
**D** True.

Note: Causes of postpartum collapse:

- Haemorrhage – may be overt or concealed (e.g. broad ligament haematoma).
- Uterine inversion is reported to cause shock which is out of proportion to blood loss, although this has been disputed.
- Pulmonary embolism.
- Uterine rupture.
- Eclampsia/epilepsy.
- CVA/MI.
- Amniotic fluid embolism.
- Vasovagal attack.

### 6.33 Answers

**A** True.
**B** True.
**C** False.
**D** True.

Note: Risk factors for postpartum haemorrhage:

- Previous PPH.
- Uterine overdistension (multiple pregnancy, polyhydramnios, macrosomia).
- High parity.
- Rapid or prolonged labour.
- Chorioamnionitis.
- APH.
- Retained products.
- Uterine anomaly/fibroids.
- Uterine trauma (rupture, scar dehiscence, inversion).
- Induction of labour.
- Operative delivery/genital tract laceration.
- General anaesthesia.
- Coagulopathy – inherited (von Willebrand's disease, haemophilia A carrier) or acquired (pre-eclampsia, liver disease, ITP).

### 6.34 Answers

**A** **True** – Thyroid dysfunction is common in the puerperium and up to 9% of women may develop disorders ranging from transient hyperthyroidism to hypothyroidism. Women with thyroid antibodies are 20x more likely to develop thyroid dysfunction.

**B** **True** – In pregnant women with ovarian cysts, torsion is most likely to occur in the puerperium.

**C** **True** – The puerperium is the most hypercoagulable phase of pregnancy and carries the highest daily risk of VTE.

**D** **True** – Post-partum psychosis usually presents 2–3 days after delivery but before 3 weeks post-partum.

**6.35 Answers**

**A False** – Breastfeeding is not contraindicated in women on antiepileptics.

**B True** – Avoiding breastfeeding is associated with a reduction in the risk of vertical transmission of HIV.

**C False.**

**D False.**

**6.36 Answers**

**A True** – Lithium is present in breast milk and risks toxicity to the infant.

**B False** – Safe in breastfeeding mothers.

**C False** – Symptoms likely to resolve earlier if breastfeeding is continued.

**D False.**

# 7. Antenatal care and fetal medicine: Questions

**7.1**    Concerning vaginal ultrasound in early pregnancy:

A The yolk sac is detected within the amniotic cavity.
B The yolk sac reaches its maximum diameter at ~12 weeks' gestation.
C The yolk sac can be detected ~35 days from the LMP.
D The fetus grows at the rate of 0.1 cm per day.

**7.2**    Concerning vaginal ultrasound in early pregnancy:

A Gestation sac volume provides a better estimate of gestation age than the crown–rump length at 7 weeks' gestation.
B The heart rate of the embryo is lowest at 9 weeks' gestation.
C In an asymptomatic woman, the finding of an empty gestation sac in the uterus is associated with a 50% risk of miscarriage.
D Cardiac activity should be detected in a viable embryo of 6 mm length.

**7.3**    Concerning vaginal ultrasound in early pregnancy:

A Absence of cardiac activity in an embryo of 3 mm reliably indicates a non-viable pregnancy.
B An intrauterine gestation sac is reliably visualized 20 days from ovulation.
C The diameter of the gestation sac grows at the rate of 1 mm per day.
D The early gestation sac is typically located in the left or right uterine cornua.

**7.4**    Nuchal translucency:

A Is more obvious at 11 weeks' than at 9 weeks' gestation.
B Is diagnostic of chromosomal anomalies.
C Is measured from the outer boarder of the cervical spine to the outer boarder of the skin.
D Is a marker of neural tube defects.

7.5     The following are typically inherited as an X-linked trait:

A Achondroplasia.
B Huntington's disease.
C Glucose-6-phosphate dehydrogenase deficiency.
D Von Willebrand's disease.


7.6     The following are typically inherited as an X-linked trait:

A Haemophilia A.
B Fragile X syndrome.
C Muscular dystrophy.
D Cystic fibrosis.


7.7     In a 30-year-old woman whose partner has haemophilia A:

A There is a 50:50 chance that her fetus has haemophilia.
B If the fetus is female, she cannot be a carrier.
C If the fetus is male, he would have haemophilia.
D Invasive procedures are absolutely contraindicated in labour unless fetal sex is known.


7.8     A child with Klinefelter's syndrome:

A Has a 46,XXY chromosomal complement.
B Has ambiguous genitalia at birth.
C Has severe intellectual impairment.
D Is fertile.


7.9     Turner's syndrome:

A Is associated with an accelerated maturation of lymphatic drainage.
B Is associated with coarctation of the aorta.
C Is associated with increasing maternal age.
D Is associated with ovarian agenesis.


7.10    Achondroplasia:

A Is the most common lethal chondrodysplasia.
B Affecting a pregnant woman is an indication for elective caesarean section.
C Is associated with learning disability.
D In a pregnant woman is associated with respiratory compromise in the third trimester.

7.11 Achondroplasia:

A Affecting a pregnant woman – epidural anaesthesia is contraindicated.
B Is more commonly due to a new mutation.
C Is caused by a mutation in the fibroblast growth factor gene.
D Is associated with increased paternal age.

7.12 Fetal alcohol syndrome:

A Is associated with an increased incidence of postmaturity.
B Seldom occurs with maternal alcohol consumption of <8 units per week.
C Is reversed by a high vitamin intake.
D Affects 1–2 per 100 000 live births.

7.13 Fetal alcohol syndrome:

A Is characteristically associated with an increased fetal abdominal circumference.
B Can be diagnosed on the basis of IUGR occurring in a woman who drinks over 20 units of alcohol per week.
C Can be diagnosed on the basis of CNS abnormalities in a woman who drinks over 20 units of alcohol per week.
D Is associated with cardiac anomalies.

7.14 Fetal hydrocephalus:

A Is associated with chromosomal anomalies in <15% of cases.
B Has a causal association with fetal viral infections.
C May be a result of the Arnold–Chiari malformation.
D Is always the result of obstruction to the flow of CSF.

7.15 Fetal hydrocephalus:

A Is associated with other major structural anomalies in <20% of cases.
B Is an indication for karyotype.
C May regress spontaneously.
D If cephalocentesis is required, it may be performed by the transabdominal or transvaginal routes.

7.16 Sacral agenesis:

A Is a recognized complication of propylthiouracil treatment in the first trimester.
B Is a recognized complication of fetal toxoplasmosis.
C Has a recognized association with elevated maternal serum AFP in mid-trimester.
D Is related to poor glucose homeostasis in the first trimester.

7.17 Anencephaly is associated with:

A Absence of the mid-brain.
B Absence of the cerebellum.
C Absence of the cerebral hemispheres.
D Adrenal hypoplasia.

7.18 Anencephaly is associated with:
A Diabetes insipidus.
B Renal agenesis.
C Anhydramnios.
D An inability of the neonate to feel pain.

7.19 With regard to neural tube defects and their detection:

A The incidence of neural tube defects is lower in insulin-dependent diabetics.
B Fetal serum AFP concentrations peak at 30 weeks' gestation.
C Maternal serum AFP concentrations fall between 15 and 18 weeks' gestation.
D Serum screening is best performed between 18–20 weeks' gestation.

7.20 Tetralogy of Fallot is characterized by:

A An atrial septal defect.
B A ventricular septal defect.
C An overriding aorta.
D Left ventricular outflow obstruction.

7.21 Trisomy 18 is associated with:

A Raised maternal serum AFP.
B Decreased maternal serum HCG.
C Decreased maternal serum unconjugated oestriol.
D Decreased nuchal thickening.

**7.22** There is a recognized association between Down syndrome and:

A Atrioventricular septal defect.
B Neonatal hypertonia.
C A chromosomal translocation defect.
D Single palmar crease.

**7.23** With respect to screening tests for Down syndrome:

A The integrated test is performed in the first trimester.
B The combined test is performed in the second trimester.
C Nuchal translucency is best measured at 10 weeks' gestation.
D The combined test does not include nuchal translucency measurement.

**7.24** With respect to Down syndrome screening:

A The combined test is more effective than the integrated test.
B The integrated test is more effective than the quadruple test.
C First trimester screening is more effective than second trimester screening.
D The integrated test is performed during the first and second trimesters.

**7.25** A 30-year-old woman requests screening for Down syndrome:

A If she is 11 weeks' pregnant, the serum integrated test should be offered.
B If nuchal translucency measurement is not available, the integrated test should be offered.
C If she specifically wants a first trimester screening test, the integrated test should be offered.
D If she is 18 weeks' pregnant, the quadruple test should be offered.

**7.26** A 30-year-old woman requests Down syndrome screening at 12 weeks' gestation:

A The integrated test is the safest test.
B The combined test is the most cost-effective test.
C Nuchal translucency measurement alone at 12–13 weeks' gestation has a 20% false-positive rate for an 85% detection rate.
D The integrated test costs £200 000 per Down syndrome pregnancy detected for an 85% detection rate.

7.27 With regards to Down syndrome due to translocation t(21:21):

A There is an increased incidence with advanced maternal age.
B The risk of an affected child is 1:2 if the mother is a balanced translocation carrier.
C It accounts for 90% of all cases of Down.
D The overall incidence is 1:700 live births.

7.28 With regards to Down syndrome due to translocation t(21;21):

A There is an increased incidence of Hirschsprung's.
B Maternal serum screening is less likely to be positive.
C The baby is likely to be mentally normal.
D The recurrence risk is lower if the mother rather than the father carries a balanced translocation.

7.29 Maternal serum AFP levels are raised in:

A The presence of closed neural tube defect.
B Fetal congenital adrenal hyperplasia.
C Exomphalos.
D Gastroschisis.

7.30 Abnormally high concentration of human chorionic gonadotrophin in pregnancy is associated with:

A Down syndrome.
B Edward syndrome.
C Intrauterine fetal death.
D Multiple pregnancy.

7.31 With regard to neural tube defects and their detection:

A Blacks have a higher incidence than Caucasians.
B Maternal serum AFP levels are higher in blacks than Caucasians.
C There is an inverse correlation between maternal serum AFP levels and maternal weight.
D Maternal serum AFP levels are higher in IDDM.

7.32 Spina bifida:

A Is associated with the Arnold–Chiari malformation.
B Should be suspected in the presence of the lemon sign on ultrasound scan.
C Should be suspected in the presence of the banana sign on ultrasound scan.
D Carries a 0.1% recurrence risk in Caucasian populations.

7.33 A 40-year-old woman whose son has been shown to have the fragile X syndrome is now 10 weeks' pregnant:

A Her affected son may have enlarged testes at puberty.
B The woman herself is no more likely to have intellectual impairment compared to the general population.
C A male fetus has a 100% chance of having the syndrome.
D A female fetus must be a carrier of the syndrome.

7.34 Chorionic villus sampling:

A Should not be performed after 20 weeks' gestation.
B If performed after 10 weeks' gestation is associated with limb reduction abnormalities.
C Should be offered after a positive first trimester screening test for Down.
D May be performed by the transabdominal or transcervical routes.

7.35 Chorionic villus sampling:

A Should be offered following positive serum screening for neural tube defects.
B Can be used in the diagnosis of trisomy 18.
C Should be offered to a woman whose partner carries a balanced translocation.
D Is contraindicated in a woman with recurrent miscarriage.

7.36 Amniocentesis performed after 16 weeks' gestation:

A Is associated with an increased risk of respiratory distress syndrome.
B Is associated with fetal postural deformities.
C Is useful in the assessment of Rhesus disease.
D Can be used to diagnose fetal infection with toxoplasmosis.

7.37  Amniocentesis performed after 16 weeks' gestation:

A  Is a definitive test in the diagnosis of fetal Down syndrome.
B  A diagnosis of chromosomal abnormality can be made within 48 hours.
C  Should not be performed after a failed CVS.
D  Trainees should perform 20 successful procedures under supervision to be deemed competent.

7.38  Antenatal fetal blood sampling:

A  Is the investigation of choice in suspected fetal hypoxia and acidosis.
B  Is contraindicated in suspected fetal thrombocytopenia.
C  May be used in the diagnosis of fetal infection.
D  Fetal blood can safely be obtained from intrahepatic vessels.

7.39  Amniocentesis is useful in the diagnosis of:

A  Tay–Sachs disease.
B  Oesophageal atresia.
C  Congenital adrenal hyperplasia.
D  Spina bifida.

7.40  Invasive testing for prenatal diagnosis should be avoided in the following circumstances:

A  In a woman who is known to carry the hepatitis B virus.
B  In a woman who is known to carry the hepatitis C virus.
C  In an HIV-positive woman with a high viral load.
D  When the transplacental route provides the only easy access to the pool of amniotic fluid.

7.41  Antenatal fetal blood sampling:

A  Is necessary for the diagnosis of fetal beta-thalassaemia.
B  Carries a 10–15% risk of premature rupture of the fetal membranes.
C  Is indicated in the investigation of fetal hydrops.
D  Has a fetal loss rate independent of indications.

7.42 Isolated renal pelvi-calyceal dilatation:

A Is associated with a five-fold increase in the risk of Down syndrome.
B Is associated with an increased risk of renal disease in postnatal life.
C Requires neonatal urological follow-up.
D Requires neonatal antibiotic prophylaxis.

7.43 With respect to soft markers for chromosomal abnormalities:

A Isolated cardiac echogenic foci are associated with an increased risk of Down syndrome.
B Fetal hyperechogenic bowel may be associated with fetal viral infection.
C The majority of fetuses with hyperechogenic bowel are normal.
D Hyperechogenic bowel is associated with an increased risk of intrauterine fetal death.

7.44 The following can be used for pre-implantation genetic diagnosis:

A Polar body from the oocyte.
B Polar body from the zygote.
C Blastomeres from cleavage stage embryos.
D Trophectoderm cells from the blastocyst.

7.45 The following can be used for pre-implantation genetic diagnosis:

A Blastocyst biopsy
B Cells from the inner cell mass
C Chorionic villus biopsy
D Amniocytes

7.46 Cleavage stage embryo biopsy for pre-implantation genetic diagnosis:

A Requires drilling of the zona pellucida.
B Is by aspiration of 3–4 blastomeres.
C Is facilitated by using culture medium supplemented with calcium and magnesium.
D Is undertaken at the 32 cell stage.

7.47 With respect to polar body biopsy for pre-implantation genetic diagnosis:

A The first polar body can be biopsied after fertilization.
B The second polar body can only be biopsied after fertilization.
C Biopsy of both polar bodies is required for accurate genetic diagnosis.
D Diagnosis of paternally derived genetic abnormalities is possible.

7.48 Pre-implantation genetic diagnosis is possible in the following conditions:

A Cystic fibrosis.
B Tay–Sachs disease.
C Beta-thalassaemia.
D Congenital adrenal hyperplasia.

7.49 Pre-implantation genetic diagnosis is possible in:

A Spinal muscular atrophy.
B Marfan's syndrome.
C Osteogenesis imperfecta.
D Fragile X syndrome.

7.50 Pre-implantation genetic diagnosis is possible in the following conditions:
A Duchenne muscular dystrophy.
B Huntington's chorea.
C Myotonic dystrophy.
D Charcot–Marie–Tooth disease.

7.51 Detection of genetic abnormalities by pre-implantation genetic diagnosis uses the following techniques:

A Cell culture and metaphase spread.
B Fluorescent in-situ hybridization.
C Polymerase chain reaction.
D Northern blotting.

7.52 The following are recognized problems when the polymerase chain reaction is used for pre-implantation genetic diagnosis:

A Allele drop-out.
B Contamination by sperm DNA.
C Contamination by DNA from laboratory personnel.
D Confined placental mosaicism.

7.53 With respect to pre-implantation genetic diagnosis:

A 1–2 cells removed from the blastocyst are representative of the rest of the embryo.
B Haploid and tetraploid nuclei are rarely found in normal human pre-implantation embryos.
C Up to 50% of normal human pre-implantation embryos show mosaicism.
D Mosaicism makes sexing of the pre-implantation embryo impossible.

7.54 Fetal haemolytic anaemia due to anti-D antibodies:

A Is secondary to intravascular haemolysis.
B Is more severe the longer the interval between the initial sensitizing event and the next pregnancy.
C Is rare when anti-D antibody levels are below 4 IU/ml.
D Is rare when anti-D antibody levels are below 10–15 IU/ml.

7.55 The following red cell antigens are not associated with fetal haemolytic disease:

A Kell antigen.
B Duffy (Fya) antigen.
C Rhesus C antigen.
D ABO antigens.

7.56 Fetal Rhesus type can be determined by:

A Amniocentesis.
B Cordocentesis.
C Analysis of fetal DNA from maternal plasma.
D Chorionic villus sampling.

7.57 In the management of pregnancy complicated by Rhesus isoimmunization:

A Paternal Rhesus zygosity can only be determined with 95% certainty.
B 56% of Rh+ fathers are heterozygous.
C Gestational age at clinical disease in a previous pregnancy is a good indicator of disease severity in the current pregnancy.
D A sinusoidal pattern on CTG is a good indicator of fetal anaemia.

7.58 Intrauterine transfusion in the treatment of Rhesus haemolytic anaemia:

A Is associated with a 3% fetal loss rate per procedure.
B Can be undertaken under fetal neuromuscular blockade with pancuronium.
C Is associated with decreased fetal cardiac output.
D Is associated with fetal acidaemia.

7.59 With respect to Rhesus D sensitization:

A The primary immune response to the D antigen occurs over 2–3 weeks.
B The primary immune response to the D antigen results in the production of IgG.
C The longer the interval between the primary D antigen challenge and a second challenge, the lower the quantity of antibody produced.
D Anti-D antibody-triggered haemolysis is complement mediated.

7.60 With regards to Rhesus disease:

A 15% of Caucasians are Rhesus positive.
B Anti-D immunoglobulin is IgM.
C Is a cause of recurrent first trimester pregnancy loss.
D Is now the commonest cause of fetal hydrops.

**7.61** In order to reduce the risk of Rhesus sensitization, it is recommended that:

A Anti-D immunoglobulin should not be given to Rhesus-positive women.

B Anti-D immunoglobulin should be given to Rhesus-negative women after a complete first trimester miscarriage.

C Anti-D should be given to Rhesus-negative women after surgical management of an ectopic pregnancy.

D In unsensitized Rhesus-negative women, blood should be taken every 4 weeks for antibody assays.

**7.62** A Rhesus-negative woman is 16 weeks into her fifth pregnancy. Her last baby had Rhesus disease requiring exchange transfusion. This pregnancy is by a new partner whose genotype is cde/CDE:

A She should be given anti-D after amniocentesis.

B Her previous partner could have been Rhesus negative.

C The current pregnancy has a 75% chance of being affected by Rhesus disease.

D If the fetus is Rhesus positive, anti-D should be given after delivery.

**7.63** A Rhesus-negative woman is 16 weeks into her fifth pregnancy. Her last baby had Rhesus disease requiring exchange transfusion. This pregnancy is by a new partner whose genotype is cde/CDE:

A A positive indirect Coombs' test performed on cord blood indicates an infant affected by Rhesus disease.

B Fetal haemoglobin concentrations can be estimated from maternal antibody concentrations.

C Maternal antibody level of 4 IU/ml should prompt cordocentesis.

D Intrauterine transfusion is recommended if severe fetal anaemia is diagnosed at 34 weeks' gestation.

**7.64** With regards to Rhesus disease:

A Affected babies are sometimes born jaundiced.

B In affected babies, erythropoiesis occurs in the fetal liver and spleen.

C Isoimmunization is more common if mother and baby are ABO incompatible.

D Bilirubin is found in the urine of affected babies.

7.65  With regards to Rhesus disease:

A Prophylactic administration of anti-D in the antenatal period significantly reduces the risk of maternal sensitization.
B Intrauterine transfusion should be with O Rh-negative blood cross-matched against maternal serum.
C Anti-C and anti-E antibodies do not cause haemolytic disease.
D The first pregnancy is never affected.

7.66  Routine antenatal anti-D prophylaxis may be unnecessary in the following circumstances:

A When the woman is known to be carrying a Rhesus-negative fetus.
B When the woman is in a stable relationship with the father of the child and he is known to be Rhesus negative.
C When the woman is certain that she would not have another child after the current pregnancy.
D When the woman has opted to be sterilized after the birth of the baby.

7.67  Intrauterine transfusion in the treatment of Rhesus haemolytic anaemia:

A Should be with Rhesus-positive packed red cells.
B Is recommended if severe anaemia is detected at 36 weeks' gestation.
C Should be performed weekly until 34 weeks' gestation.
D Is not necessary if fetal haematocrit is >30%.

7.68  The following condition is characteristically associated with oligo-hydramnios:

A Talipes equinovarus.
B Fetal imperforate anus.
C Fetal congenital adrenal hyperplasia.
D Anencephaly.

7.69  Oligohydramnios is characteristically associated with:
A Diabetes mellitus.
B Rhesus disease.
C Fetal renal agenesis.
D Placental haemangioma.

7.70   Oligohydramnios is characteristically associated with:

   A  IUGR.
   B  Fetal duodenal atresia.
   C  Hirschprung's disease.
   D  Multiple pregnancy.


7.71   The following congenital anomalies are associated with oligohydramnios:

   A  Juvenile polycystic kidney disease.
   B  Unilateral renal agenesis.
   C  Duodenal atresia.
   D  Posterior urethral valves.


7.72   A 24-year-old woman is found to have idiopathic polyhydramnios at 30 weeks' gestation. The following treatments may improve fetal outcome:

   A  Indomethacin.
   B  Sulindac.
   C  Betamethasone.
   D  Insulin.


7.73   Polyhydramnios is characteristically associated with:

   A  Polycystic kidney disease.
   B  Imperforate anus.
   C  Fetal congenital adrenal hyperplasia.
   D  Congenital diaphragmatic hernia.


7.74   With regards to twin pregnancy:

   A  Perinatal mortality is reduced.
   B  Maternal mortality is significantly increased.
   C  Monozygotic twins have a similar incidence worldwide.
   D  Dizygotic twins are more common.


7.75   In twin pregnancies:

   A  Monozygotic twins are always identical.
   B  Monochorionic twins are always identical.
   C  Dichorionic twins may be identical.
   D  Discordant growth should be diagnosed when there is a discrepancy of >10% in estimated weight.

7.76 With regard to twin pregnancy:

A Polyhydramnios is more common.
B Oligohydramnios is more common.
C Caesarean section is recommended if the first twin is breech.
D The second twin should be delivered by caesarean section if in a breech presentation.

7.77 With regards to twin pregnancies:

A Postpartum haemorrhage is less common.
B Induction of labour is contraindicated.
C Intrapartum intermittent auscultation is acceptable management.
D An abnormal fetal heart pattern in twin 2 should prompt fetal blood sampling.

7.78 With regards to multiple pregnancy:

A Corticosteroids are recommended from 30 weeks' gestation.
B Tocolysis is absolutely contraindicated.
C Down syndrome is more common.
D Congenital anomalies are less common.

7.79 Gastroschisis:

A Is a normal finding before 13 weeks' gestation.
B Is associated with chromosomal abnormalities and a karyotype is recommended.
C Vaginal delivery is contraindicated.
D Is associated with sudden unexplained fetal death.

7.80 An exomphalos:

A Is covered by skin.
B Is a persistence of physiological herniation of the bowel.
C Is associated with raised maternal serum AFP.
D Is associated with chromosomal anomalies.

7.81 A fetal karyotype is indicated in the presence of the following anomalies:
A Duodenal atresia.
B Gastroschisis.
C Exomphalos.
D Atrioventricular septal defect.

7.82 A 30-year-old woman is found to have a hydropic fetus at 25 weeks' gestation. The following are possible causes:

A Parvovirus B19 infection.
B Bilateral renal agenesis.
C Rhesus disease.
D Duodenal atresia.

7.83 The following investigations are relevant in the investigation of the hydropic fetus:

A Fetal blood sampling.
B Syphilis serology.
C Kleihauer test.
D Maternal blood group.

7.84 There is a recognized association between intrauterine death of the fetus and:

A Maternal CMV infection.
B Sickle cell trait.
C Listeriosis.
D Gestational diabetes mellitus.

7.85 The biophysical profile:

A A score of 8 is always normal.
B Perinatal mortality rises with a falling score.
C Makes use of umbilical artery Dopplers.
D Is of no use after 37 weeks' gestation.

7.86 Spontaneous preterm labour:

A Is a recognized complication of cryo-cautery to the cervix.
B Is a recognized complication of cone biopsy.
C Is more common in women with a previous preterm delivery.
D Is more common in women with a history of antepartum haemorrhage.

7.87 Spontaneous preterm labour:

A Is associated with low maternal weight at booking.
B Is associated with maternal smoking.
C Is more common in teenage pregnancy.
D Without preterm rupture of membranes should not be treated with antibiotics.

7.88 The following are risk factors for spontaneous preterm delivery:

A Threatened miscarriage.
B Antepartum haemorrhage.
C Vaginal candidiasis.
D Previous preterm delivery.

7.89 The following are risk factors for spontaneous preterm delivery:

A Maternal obesity.
B Smoking.
C Asymptomatic bacteriuria.
D Working with visual display units.

7.90 The following drugs have a tocolytic effect:

A Magnesium sulphate.
B Salbutamol.
C Indomethacin.
D Aspirin.

7.91 The following drugs have been shown to have a tocolytic effect:

A Ritodrine.
B Terbutaline.
C Misoprostol.
D Mifepristone.

7.92 The following drugs have a tocolytic effect:

A Ethanol.
B Nimesulide.
C Nifedipine.
D Atosiban.

7.93 The use of intravenous ritodrine on its own is associated with:

A Reduced fetal movements.
B A reduction in preterm delivery rate.
C A reduction in perinatal morbidity.
D A reduction in perinatal mortality.

7.94 The administration of corticosteroids to women in preterm labour is associated with:

A Increased maternal mortality.
B Decreased maternal morbidity.
C Reduced infant growth.
D Decreased perinatal mortality.

7.95 The following are relative contraindications to the use of antenatal corticosteroids:

A Maternal tuberculosis.
B Maternal urinary tract infection.
C Imminent preterm delivery.
D Maternal prednisolone therapy.

7.96 The administration of corticosteroids to women in preterm labour is associated with:
A Decreased risk of intraventricular haemorrhage.
B Increased risk of pulmonary hypertension.
C Decreased risk of preterm delivery.
D Increased risk of chorioamnionitis.

7.97 A 20-year-old woman presents at 20 weeks' gestation with ruptured membranes:

A Corticosteroids should be administered.
B Tocolytics should be administered if uterine activity is detected.
C Infection is a likely aetiological factor.
D If the pregnancy progresses to 27 weeks' gestation, pulmonary hypoplasia is unlikely.

7.98 A 20-year-old woman presents at 20 weeks' gestation with ruptured membranes:

A Termination of pregnancy should be recommended.
B In the presence of vaginal Group B streptococcal colonization, termination of pregnancy should be recommended.
C In the presence of maternal pyrexia, termination of pregnancy should be recommended.
D Postural deformities are a potential fetal complication.

**7.99** Pre-labour rupture of the membranes:

A Occurring at 25 weeks' gestation – perinatal morbidity is reduced by treatment with erythromycin.

B Occurring at 25 weeks' gestation – perinatal morbidity is reduced by treatment with augmentin.

C May be due to intrinsic weakness in the membranes.

D Can be managed with cervical cerclage at 25 weeks' gestation.

**7.100** A 34-year-old primigravida presents with abdominal pain and uterine contractions at 33 weeks' gestation:

A Corticosteroids should be administered.

B Tocolytics should be administered.

C Erythromycin should be prescribed.

D The presence of a normal fetal heart rate excludes a concealed abruption.

**7.101** A 34-year-old primigravida presents with abdominal pain and uterine contractions at 33 weeks' gestation:

A The presence of constant abdominal pain is suggestive of a concealed abruption.

B A normal placental site scan excludes placental abruption.

C The membranes should be ruptured if the cervix is unchanged after 4 hours of regular painful contractions.

D A Kleihauer test may be useful if placental abruption is suspected.

**7.102** Fetal fibronectin:

A Is produced by the decidua.

B Is a glycoprotein.

C Has a high sensitivity in predicting delivery within 10 days in women symptomatic of preterm labour.

D Is useful in predicting delivery before 34 weeks in asymptomatic women.

**7.103** The following drugs and side effects are associated:

A Nifedipine and hypertension.

B Ritodrine and hyperkalaemia.

C Indomethacin and oligohydramnios.

D Magnesium sulphate and apnoea.

7.104 The following drugs and side effects are associated:

A Magnesium sulphate and hyperglycaemia.
B Atosiban and fluid retention.
C Ritodrine and fetal tachycardia.
D Nifedipine and headache.

7.105 The following are relative contraindications to the use of antenatal corticosteroids:

A Multiple pregnancy.
B Maternal insulin-dependent diabetes mellitus.
C Preterm premature rupture of membranes.
D Suspected chorioamnionitis.

7.106 With respect to breech presentation:

A The risk of significant congenital abnormality at 30 weeks' gestation is <5%.
B Male infants are at greater risk of congenital dislocation of the hip than female infants.
C The incidence is greater with delivery at 30 weeks' than at 38 weeks' gestation.
D Congenital hip dislocation is unrelated to the mode of delivery.

7.107 With respect to breech presentation:

A ECV carried out at 36 weeks' gestation significantly reduces the incidence of breech presentation at term.
B ECV should be preceded by an ultrasound scan.
C ECV is contraindicated when there has been antepartum haemorrhage of any cause.
D ECV should only be undertaken in conjunction with the use of tocolytics.

7.108 With respect to breech presentation:

A ECV is more likely to be successful in Caucasian than in black African women.
B Meta-analysis has shown that caesarean section is the optimal mode of delivery before term.
C Regardless of mode of delivery, neonatal mortality and morbidity are higher at a given gestational age than with cephalic presentation.
D 10% of fetuses with hydrocephalus present by breech position.

7.109 With respect to breech presentation:

A There is an association with oligohydramnios.
B There is an increased feto-placental ratio.
C There is an increased head circumference regardless of mode of delivery.
D There is an association with a short umbilical cord.

**7.1    Answers**

**A** False.

**B** **False** – Maximum yolk sac diameter reached ~10 weeks (6 mm). Yolk sac is compressed against the wall of the chorionic cavity by the expanding amniotic cavity and is not detectable after 12 weeks.

**C** **True** – First detectable on TV scan at ~35 days from LMP at 3–4 mm diameter.

**D** **True** – Embryo grows at ~1 mm per day.

**7.2    Answers**

**A** **False** – The biological variability of CRL is small and growth is rapid – it is therefore the most accurate ultrasound estimate of gestational age. In multiple pregnancies, the larger CRL should be used for assigning gestational age.

**B** **False** – Embryonic heart rate increases between 6 and 9 weeks, followed by a slight decline after 10 weeks.

**C** **False** – In asymptomatic women, the risk of miscarriage is 12% when an empty gestation sac is identified by ultrasound, 7.2% when a live embryo with CRL <5 mm is detected, 3.3% for embryos of 6–10 mm and 0.5% when a live embryo with CRL >10 mm is detected.

**D** **True** – All viable embryos with CRL >7 mm should demonstrate cardiac activity.

Note:

* The embryo is detectable at ~37 days from LMP by TV scan as a bright linear echo adjacent to the yolk sac. CRL ~2 mm and cardiac activity can be identified.

**7.3    Answers**

**A** **False** – See 7.2D.

**B** **True** – The gestation sac is the first pregnancy structure that can be detected – usually visualized at 31 days from the LMP using transvaginal scanning and measures 2–3 mm in diameter. Detectable by transabdominal scanning at ~5 + 3 weeks' gestation.

**C** **True.**

**D** **False** – Typically centrally located within the fundus.

### 7.4 Answers

**A** **True** – Nuchal translucency increases with gestational age to peak at 13 + 2, after which it decreases. Optimum gestational age for first trimester scan is 13 weeks.

**B** **False** – Risk of trisomy 21 increases with increased NT from 3 mm (three-fold increase in maternal age-related risk) to >6 mm (36-fold increase in risk). The presence of septations increases the risk of aneuploidy. Risk of aneuploidy may be up to 32% with an abnormal NT. Increased NT also associated with Turner's syndrome, Noonan's syndrome, Robert's syndrome.

**C** **False** – Measured by placing the intersection of the calipers on the outer boarder of the cervical spine and the inner boarder of the skin lying directly posterior to it.

**D** **True** – Increased NT associated with structural anomalies, in particular cardiac (ventricular and atrioventricular septal defects and narrowing of the aortic isthmus), omphalocele, and anencephaly. There is also an association with fetal loss and perinatal mortality.

Note:
* In the second trimester, nuchal translucency is considered abnormal if >5 mm after 15 weeks' gestation.

### 7.5 Answers

**A** False.
**B** False.
**C** True.
**D** False.

Note:
* X-linked traits: Alport syndrome, androgen insensitivity syndrome, colour blindness, Fabry disease, glucose-6-phosphate dehydrogenase deficiency, haemophilia A/B, Lesch–Nyhan syndrome, muscular dystrophy – Duchenne/Becker, fragile X syndrome.

### 7.6 Answers

**A** True.
**B** **True** – Males affected almost exclusively, transmitted from carrier females to their sons, affected males cannot transmit the disorder to their sons.
**C** True.
**D** **False** – Cystic fibrosis is autosomal recessive.

## 7.7 Answers

**A  False** – X-linked recessive disorder – only males affected although carrier females may have abnormally low Factor VIII levels and a bleeding tendency due to Lyonization.

**B  False** – Female fetuses will all be carriers as they would have inherited the defective X chromosome from their father.

**C  False** – All male fetuses will be unaffected as they inherit the Y chromosome from their father.

**D  False** – As there is no risk of an affected fetus, there is no indication for modifying care.

## 7.8 Answers

**A  False** – 47,XXY.

**B  False** – Diagnosis typically made following infertility investigation – commonest cause of hypogonadism and infertility in males. Poorly developed secondary sexual characteristics, small testicles, gynaecomastia, increased height (elongated limbs).

**C  False** – IQ 10–20 points lower than siblings.

**D  False** – Infertility is universal except in mosaics.

Note:

- Incidence 1:1000 males; risk increases with increased maternal age.
- Extra X chromosome is maternal in 50–60% of cases; recurrence risk close to population risk.
- Low testosterone levels.
- Gynaecomastia with increased risk of breast cancer.
- Associated with increased risk of diabetes mellitus, osteoporosis, scoliosis and emphysema.
- Testosterone replacement at puberty/adulthood to promote development of secondary sexual characteristics.

## 7.9 Answers

**A  False.**

**B  True** – Associated with increased nuchal transluscency, coarctation of the aorta, atrial septal defects, cystic hygroma, fetal hydrops.

**C  False** – Associated with young maternal age.

**D  False** – Streak ovaries with primary amenorrhoea (ovarian dysgenesis).

Note:

- 45X0.
- There is short stature with no adolescent growth spurt, webbed neck, wide carrying angle, hypoplasia of the nails and short fourth metacarpals, broad chest with widely spaced nipples and a low hair line; associated with peripheral lymphoedema in 40% of cases.
- Increased risk of systemic hypertension and Hashimoto's thyroiditis.
- Normal intellectual development.

### 7.10 Answers

**A** False.
**B** True – Women with achondroplasia should be delivered by caesarean section because of narrowing of the pelvis.
**C** False.
**D** True.

Note:
- Children affected with achondroplasia frequently have delayed motor milestones, otitis media, and bowing of the knees. Occasionally, in infancy or early childhood, there is symptomatic airway obstruction, development of thoracolumbar kyphosis, symptomatic hydrocephalus, or symptomatic upper cord compression.

### 7.11 Answers

**A** True – General anaesthaesia is usually required.
**B** True – 75% of individuals are born to parents of average height – new mutations.
**C** False – Autosomal dominant – mutation on the fibroblast growth factor receptor III gene located on chromosome 4.
**D** True – Older fathers (>40 years) are more likely to have a child with achondroplasia (and other autosomal dominant conditions) secondary to a new mutation.

### 7.12 Answers

**A** False.
**B** True – Occurs in 30–33% of women consuming ~18 units of alcohol/day. Fetal susceptibility may be dependent on the presence of other factors including smoking, nutrition, drug use and social deprivation.
**C** False.
**D** False – 1–2 per 1000 live births.

### 7.13 Answers

**A** False.
**B** False – Diagnosis requires signs in all of the three following categories: (1) IUGR; (2) CNS involvement (neurological abnormalities, developmental delay, intellectual impairment, head circumference below the third centile, brain malformation); (3) characteristic facial deformity (short palpebral fissures, elongated mid-face, flattened maxilla).
**C** False – See B.
**D** True – Other associated anomalies include cardiac anomalies (ASD and VSD), optic nerve hypoplasia, poor visual acuity, hearing loss, renal hypoplasia, bladder diverticulae and skeletal deformities.

## 7.14 Answers

**A** **True** – 10% have chromosomal anomaly, therefore offer karyotype.
**B** **True.**
**C** **True.**
**D** **False** – Typically classified as obstructive (non-communicating hydrocephalus), communicating hydrocephalus (over-production of CSF, impaired resorption) or deficiency of cortical tissue with relative increase in ventricular size (hydrocephalus ex vacuo). Obstructive causes are commonest in fetus/neonate.

Note:

- Fetal hydrocephalus is ventriculomegaly causing enlargement of the head.
- Meningomyelocele is the most common anomaly associated with hydrocephalus.
- Causes: malformation of CNS structures – hereditary hydrocephalus or hydrocephalus associated with a malformation syndrome including the Arnold–Chiari malformation; in utero infection; intraventricular haemorrhage; intracranial tumours/mass lesions.

## 7.15 Answers

**A** **False** – 59–85% have other major anomaly.
**B** **True** – See 7.14A.
**C** **True.**
**D** **True** – 14–22 gauge needle transabdominally or transvaginally.

Note: Management of fetal hydrocephalus:

- Explain anomaly and prognosis.
- Screen for other anomalies including cardiac and meningomyelocele.
- Offer karyotype.
- Screen for infection.
- Offer TOP.
- If pregnancy is continued, serial scans – few cases of spontaneous regression.
- Discuss risks and benefits of ventriculo-amniotic shunts in a tertiary centre.
- If progressive, aim for delivery once fetus is mature to limit consequences of ventricular enlargement. Vaginal delivery appropriate if mild macrocephaly.
- If associated with anomalies with a poor prognosis, cephalocentesis. Destructive procedure associated with ~90% perinatal death.
- Counsel about recurrence risk, especially if hereditary hydrocephalus (various sex-linked recessive and autosomal dominant variants reported).

## 7.16 Answers

**A** **False.**
**B** **False.**
**C** **False.**
**D** **True** – Associated with maternal insulin-dependent diabetes (16–50%).

Note:

- Developmental disorders of the lower portions of the spinal column and pelvis.
- Incidence ~1 in 25 000 children.
- Girls and boys are affected equally.
- Associated with monozygotic twins.
- Associated with urogenital and anorectal anomalies.
- Karyotype recommended as similar abnormalities may be associated with chromosomal anomalies.

### 7.17 Answers

**A** False.

**B** True.

**C** True.

**D** True – There is pituitary hypoplasia leading to diabetes insipidus and adrenal hypoplasia secondary to absent ACTH.

Note:

- Cephalic end of the neural tube fails to close. Absence of the forebrain, including cerebral hemispheres, skull and scalp. The remaining brain tissue is often exposed. A rudimentary brainstem may be present.
- Incidence falling. Higher in Caucasian population compared to African/Asian. Higher in Wales/Ireland.

### 7.18 Answers

**A** True – See 7.17D.

**B** False.

**C** False.

**D** True – The infant is usually blind, deaf, unconscious and unable to feel pain.

Note:

- Reflex actions such as respiration and responses to sound or touch may occur.
- Associated with cleft palate, cardiac anomalies and polyhydramnios.
- Stillbirth or death shortly after birth.
- Use of organs for transplantation is controversial.

### 7.19 Answers

**A** False – IDDM is a risk factor for neural tube defects.

**B** False.

**C** False – Maternal serum concentrations peak at ~30–32 weeks' gestation and rise linearly between 15 and 20 weeks.

**D** False – Serum screening best performed at 15–20 weeks.

Note: Risk factors for neural tube defects:

- Family history (including third-degree relations; 2–5% risk if one affected child, 1–5% risk if parent affected).
- IDDM.
- Antiepileptic therapy.
- Gastric bypass surgery.

## 7.20 Answers

**A** False.
**B** True.
**C** True.
**D** False.

Note:

- 0.4 per 1000 live births.
- Ventricular septal defect, right ventricular outflow obstruction (pulmonary infundibular stenosis), overriding aorta, right ventricular hypertrophy.
- Baby pink at birth, becomes cyanosed with crying or feeding – cyanosis develops and progresses over the first few weeks of life.
- Cyanosis occurs at rest in childhood with 'squatting' behaviour – traps venous blood in legs, increases resistance in aorta, hence reducing right-to-left shunt.
- 95% survival after corrective surgery.

## 7.21 Answers

**A** False – Associated with low maternal serum AFP.
**B** True.
**C** True.
**D** False – Associated with increasd nuchal translucency.

Note:

- 1:8000 live births; 95% of conceptions with trisomy 18 spontaneously miscarry. Two-thirds of fetuses diagnosed by second-trimester amniocentesis spontaneously miscarry.
- 10% of live births survive first year with profound developmental delay.
- Associated with multiple anomalies including: early-onset IUGR, rockerbottom feet, clenched fist, overlapping fingers, choroid plexus cyst, two vessel cord, increased nuchal transluscency, oligohydramnios, polyhydramnios, renal/cardiac/CNS/skeletal anomalies.

## 7.22 Answers

**A** True – 55% of neonates with Down syndrome have a structural anomaly – cardiac anomalies (atrioventricular canal defects), GI (duodenal atresia, exomphalos, Hirschprung disease), urinary tract, limb defects (fifth finger clinodactily), congenital cataract.
**B** False – Neonatal hypotonia.
**C** True.
**D** True.

Note:

- Severe learning disability.
- Brachycephaly, upslanting palpebral fissures, Brushfield spots, epicanthic folds, open mouth with protruding tongue.
- Increased risk of leukaemia, thyroid disease, Alzheimer's, epilepsy.
- Life expectancy 50–55 years.

### 7.23 Answers

**A** **False** – Integrated test: NT and PAPP-A at 10 completed weeks' gestation + AFP, free beta-HCG, uE3 and inhibin-A at 14–20 weeks' gestation.

**B** **False** – Combined test: NT, free beta-HCG and PAPP-A at 10 completed weeks' gestation.

**C** **False** – NT measurement best at 12–13 completed weeks' gestation.

**D** **False** – See B.

### 7.24 Answers

**A** **False** – Integrated test is most effective screening test with a false-positive rate of 1.2% (1.0–1.4) for an 85% detection rate. Combined test has a 6.1% (5.6–6.5) false-positive rate for an 85% detection rate.

**B** **True** – See A. Quadruple test (AFP, uE3, free beta-HCG and inhibin-A at 14–20 weeks' gestation) has a 6.2% (5.8–6.6) false-positive rate for an 85% detection rate.

**C** **False** – First trimester screening is as effective as second trimester screening and both are less effective than integrated screening.

**D** **True** – See 7.23A.

### 7.25 Answers

**A** **False** – At 11 weeks, the integrated test should be offered.

**B** **False** – The integrated test includes NT – if this is not available, the serum integrated test should be offered.

**C** **False** – The integrated test involves testing in the first and second trimester. See 7.23A.

**D** **True** – The quadruple test is the most effective second trimester test.

### 7.26 Answers

**A** **True** – Integrated test – 9 diagnostic-procedure-related pregnancy losses per 100 000 women screened for an 85% detection rate. Equivalent figure for combined test is 44 pregnancy losses and for quadruple test is 45 pregnancy losses.

**B** **False** – For an 85% detection rate, the cost in the UK per Down syndrome fetus detected would be £15 300 for the integrated test, £16 800 for the quadruple test and £19 000 for the combined test.

**C** **True.**

**D** **False** – See B.

## 7.27 Answers

**A** False.

**B** False – No translocation – age-related risk + 0.34% at term (0.42% mid-trimester).

**C** False – 95% due to trisomy 21, 4% due to translocation involving chromosome 21, 1% mosaic. Extra chromosome 21 of maternal origin in ~90% of cases – mostly due to non-dysjunction in first meiotic division.

**D** False – Incidence of Down syndrome is ~1:700 live births.

## 7.28 Answers

**A** True – Associated with Hirschprung's disease.

**B** False – No evidence that serum screening efficacy is affected by aetiology of the syndrome.

**C** False.

**D** False – Mother carrier of t(14:21) – 15% recurrence risk, father carrier of t(14:21) – 1% recurrence risk, mother or father t(21:21) – 100% recurrence risk.

## 7.29 Answers

**A** False.

**B** False.

**C** True.

**D** True.

Note: Other causes of raised MSAFP:
- Wrong dates (under-estimation), multiple pregnancy, abdominal wall defects, upper GI obstruction, congenital nephrosis, placental/cord tumour, obstructive uropathy, feto-maternal haemorrhage, CAML (cystic adenomatoid malformation of the lung), sacrococcyteal teratoma, maternal liver disease, smoking, Afro-Caribbean ethnic background.
- Male fetus.

## 7.30 Answers

**A** True.

**B** False – HCG levels are low in Edward syndrome.

**C** False.

**D** True.

Note:
- Raised HCG levels are associated with Down syndrome, multiple pregnancy, molar pregnancy and wrong dates.

## 7.31 Answers

**A** **False** – Risk of NTD is lower in Blacks than Caucasians.
**B** **True.**
**C** **True.**
**D** **False.**

Note:
- Low MSAFP with wrong dates (over-estimation), high maternal weight, Down syndrome, trisomy 18, IDDM.

## 7.32 Answers

**A** **True** – Associated with the Arnold–Chiari malformation in 90–95% of cases: caudal displacement of the cerebellar vermis and medulla and fourth ventricle. This leads to: *lemon sign* – scalloping of frontal bones due to caudal displacement of cranial content, and *banana sign* – flattened cerebellar hemispheres with obliteration of the cisterna magna; flow of CSF is eventually obstructed and hydrocephalus develops.
**B** **True.**
**C** **True.**
**D** **False** – Recurrence risk is 1–5%.

Note:
- Prognosis dependent on level and length of defect and presence of neural tissue in meningeal sac.
- Counsel regarding recurrence risk and recommend pre-conception folic acid (5 mg) for subsequent pregnancy.

## 7.33 Answers

**A** **True** – Males with the full mutation have enlarged testes after puberty (50%).
**B** **False** – Females with the full mutation may be normal or have mild or moderate learning disability. Prediction of degree of mental impairment is not possible prenatally. Males with the full mutation have learning difficulty.
**C** **False.**
**D** **False.**

Note:
- Fragile site at Xq27.3 under culture conditions with thymidine or deoxycytidine deprivation.
- Males/females with the pre-mutation are normal. The length of the pre-mutation is however unstable and expansion at meiosis to the full mutation is possible (risk of expansion increases with increasing length of the pre-mutation).
- Prenatal diagnosis by DNA analysis (CVS or amniocentesis).

## 7.34 Answers

**A** **False** – CVS may be undertaken safely at any gestational age after 10 weeks.

**B** **False** – If performed before 10 weeks is associated with fetal limb reduction abnormalities.

**C** **True** – Investigation of choice after positive first trimester screening.

**D** **True** – Transcervical CVS (first trimester) appears to be associated with a small increase in fetal loss rate compared to second trimester amniocentesis. There does not appear to be a difference between transabdominal CVS and second trimester amniocentesis with respect to fetal loss.

## 7.35 Answers

**A** **False** – Positive serum screening for neural tube defects should be investigated by ultrasound scan or amniocentesis.

**B** **True** – Used in the diagnosis of aneuploidy and chromosomal translocations.

**C** **True.**

**D** **False** – A history of recurrent miscarriage is not a contraindication to CVS.

## 7.36 Answers

**A** **False** – Amniocentesis performed after 15 weeks is not associated with increased risk of respiratory distress or postural deformities; this may be the case with early amniocentesis (before 15 weeks).

**B** **False.**

**C** **True** – Although amniocentesis may be used in the management of Rhesus disease, most current management involves ultrasound-based fetal assessment with fetal blood sampling.

**D** **True** – Amniocentesis + PCR may be used to diagnose fetal infection.

## 7.37 Answers

**A** **True** – Definitive diagnostic test for fetal aneuploidy.

**B** **True** – Results may be available within 48 hours using FISH.

**C** **False** – Can be undertaken after failed CVS.

**D** **False** – There is no longer a recommended number of procedures that should be performed before competence is determined.

## 7.38 Answers

**A** **False** – In suspected fetal hypoxia/acidosis, biophysical methods of fetal assessment should be used. PH may be measured following fetal blood sampling but suspected acidosis is not an indication for antenatal FBS.

**B** **False** – FBS is used to guide diagnosis and treatment of fetal thrombocytopenia.

**C** **True** – FBS + PCR would be the gold standard to confirm fetal infection, although this does not provide information on the severity of any consequent impairment.

**D** **True** – Fetal blood may be obtained from umbilical cord vessels, fetal heart and intrahepatic vessels.

### 7.39 Answers

**A True** – Tay–Sachs disease is an autosomal recessive condition secondary to hexosaminidase A deficiency. Prenatal diagnosis by amniocentesis is possible.

**B False.**

**C True** – Prenatal diagnosis by amniocentesis or CVS is possible for CAH secondary to 21-hydroxylase deficiency.

**D True** – Amniotic fluid AFP and cholinesterase concentrations are useful in the diagnosis of spina bifida. Spina bifida occulta, however, is not detectable by analysis of amniotic fluid.

### 7.40 Answers

**A False** – Invasive testing may be performed in carriers of hepatitis B and C. The available evidence is that the risk of transmission is low.

**B False.**

**C True** – Testing should be avoided in HIV-positive women, especially in the third trimester.

**D False** – The transplacental route should be avoided but may be used if it provides the only easy access to the pool of liquor.

### 7.41 Answers

**A False** – The beta chain is not present in fetal Hb – single gene defects can be diagnosed by amniocentesis or CVS.

**B False** – Risk of membrane rupture with FBS is small and similar to that with amniocentesis.

**C True.**

**D False** – Procedure-related fetal loss – 0–2.5% (average ~1%), higher risk if transfusion performed. Risk of fetal loss is related to indication for FBS – 25% for non-immune hydrops, 1.5% for prenatal diagnosis.

Note:

• FBS is the definitive test for the diagnosis of fetal anaemia.

### 7.42 Answers

**A False** – Association with aneuploidy is very small and karyotype is not indicated.

**B True.**

**C True** – Identifies fetuses requiring postnatal urological assessment (renal scan at about 1 week of age) + prophylactic antibiotics.

**D True.**

Note:

• Antero-posterior diameter of the renal pelvis >4 mm before 33 weeks' gestation and >7 mm thereafter.

### 7.43 Answers

**A** **False** – Karyotype not indicated for isolated cardiac echogenic foci. Most resolve spontaneously.
**B** **True** – See D.
**C** **True** – This is a physiological variant in most cases.
**D** **True** – There is an association with cystic fibrosis, meconium ileus, trisomy 21, CMV infection, IUGR and intrauterine death.

Note:
- Cardiac echogenic foci – hyperechogenicity is thought to be attached to the chordae tendinae, not to the ventricular walls and moving simultaneously with the atrioventricular valves.
- Hyperechogenic bowel is a subjective assessment; diagnosis is made when the echogenicity of fetal bowel is similar to or greater than that of surrounding bone.

### 7.44 Answers

**A** **True.**
**B** **True.**
**C** **True.**
**D** **True** – However, up to 60% of human embryos arrest in culture and do not reach the blastocyst stage. Blastocyst biopsy gives more cells for diagnosis but less time as the blastocyst would have to be transferred into the uterus as soon as possible.

Note:
- Most centres use cleavage stage embryo biopsy.

### 7.45 Answers

**A** **False.**
**B** **False.**
**C** **False.**
**D** **False.**

### 7.46 Answers

**A** **True** – Zona drilling may be performed using acid Tyrodes solution, laser or partial zona dissection.
**B** **False** – 1–2 blastomeres are aspirated after drilling of the zona pellucida.
**C** **False** – Compaction of the embryo begins to occur after the 8-cell stage with the formation of intercellular junctions – this is $Ca^{2+}/Mg^{2+}$ dependent. Biopsy is therefore facilitated by using $Ca^{2+}/Mg^{2+}$-free culture medium.
**D** **False** – Undertaken at the 8–10 cell stage, 3 days after fertilization.

## 7.47 Answers

**A** True.

**B** True – Second polar body is only released after fertilization.

**C** True – Removal of both polar bodies is required for accurate diagnosis. Can be performed simultaneously or sequentially.

**D** False – Only maternal chromosomes are examined.

Note:

- Used in the diagnosis of common aneuploidies in IVF.

## 7.48 Answers

**A** True.

**B** True.

**C** True.

**D** True.

## 7.49 Answers

**A** True.

**B** True.

**C** True.

**D** True.

## 7.50 Answers

**A** True.

**B** True.

**C** True.

**D** True.

Note:

- Pre-implantation genetic diagnosis is currently possible in the following conditions. The number of conditions is however constantly increasing: cystic fibrosis, Tay–Sachs disease, beta-thalassaemia, congenital adrenal hyperplasia, spinal muscular atrophy, Marfan's syndrome, osteogenesis imperfecta, fragile X syndrome, Duchenne muscular dystrophy, Huntington's chorea, myotonic dystrophy, Charcot–Marie–Tooth disease, familial adenomatous polyposis coli, retinitis pigmentosum.

## 7.51 Answers

**A** False – Pre-implantation diagnosis uses a single cell for diagnosis. This is made possible by the use of PCR technology, amplifying fragments of DNA thousands of times.

**B** True – FISH uses fluorescent tagged DNA probes that bind to specific DNA sequences.

**C** True – See A.

**D** False.

## 7.52    Answers

**A** **True** – Allele drop-out is the preferential amplification of one allele only and is particularly important in autosomal dominant conditions. If the mutated allele drops out, the embryo would be erroneously diagnosed as normal.

**B** **True** – Contamination by DNA from the environment, laboratory staff and other cells, including sperm and cumulus cells.

**C** **True** – For this reason, intracytoplasmic sperm injection (ICSI) is used prior to pre-implantation genetic diagnosis.

**D** **False** – Confined placental mosaicism is encountered during CVS.

## 7.53    Answers

**A** **False** – It is now recognized that 1–2 cells biopsied from the blastocyst are not necessarily representative of the rest of the embryo.

**B** **False.**

**C** **True** – Up to 50% of human pre-implantation embryos show mosaicism, the commonest abnormalities being haploid and tetraploid nuclei.

**D** **False** – Mosaicism does not affect sexing as female cells would have to appear in a male embryo (or vice versa).

## 7.54    Answers

**A** **False** – Anti-D antibody coated red cells undergo extravascular destruction by the reticuloendothelial system.

**B** **True** – The longer the interval between exposures the higher the quantity of antibody produced and the better the binding of the antibody to red cells; this increases the risk of severe fetal disease.

**C** **True** – Significant fetal anaemia is not expected when the anti-D titre remains below 1:64. Severe fetal anaemia is not expected at anti-D levels below 4 IU/ml.

**D** **True** – Severe fetal anaemia is rare below 10–15 IU/ml.

## 7.55    Answers

**A** **False.**

**B** **False** – Kidd and Duffy antigens are uncommon causes of fetal haemolytic disease.

**C** **False** – Antigens that commonly cause fetal haemolytic disease include Rhesus antigens D, C, E, c, e and Kell antigens.

**D** **True.**

Note:

- Maternal red cell alloimmunization results from exposure to foreign red cell antigens.

### 7.56 Answers

**A** True.
**B** True.
**C** True.
**D** True.

Note:
- Paternal zygosity and fetal typing can be determined using PCR technology with paternal blood/amniocentesis or CVS. Fetal typing may also be undertaken using fetal DNA from maternal plasma – repeat testing is recommended in the case of a Rh-negative result. The fetus can only be affected if it is Rh-positive.

### 7.57 Answers

**A** False – Paternal zygosity can be determined with certainty using PCR technology and paternal blood.
**B** True.
**C** False – Severity of disease increases with parity. Obstetric history, and in particular gestational age at clinical disease in a previous pregnancy, is a poor predictor of disease.
**D** False – CTG sinusoidal pattern is rare, even in severe fetal anaemia.

### 7.58 Answers

**A** True – Intrauterine transfusion is associated with a procedure-related fetal loss rate of 2–4%.
**B** True – May be facilitated by fetal neuromuscular blockade.
**C** True – Treatment of anaemia results in decreased cardiac output.
**D** True – Transfusion of packed red cells is associated with acidaemia.

### 7.59 Answers

**A** False – The primary response to the D antigen is usually weak, occurs over 6 weeks–12 months.
**B** False – The primary response is mainly an IgM response (does not cross the placenta).
**C** False – The response following a second antigenic challenge is rapid and mainly an IgG response. The longer the interval between exposures the higher the quantity of antibody produced and the better the binding of the antibody to red cells – the risk of severe fetal disease is increased.
**D** False – see 7.54A.

**7.60    Answers**

    **A  False** – 15% of Caucasians are Rh negative.
    **B  False** – Anti-D immunoglobulin is IgG and therefore crosses the placenta.
    **C  False** – Rhesus disease does not cause recurrent first trimester pregnancy loss as the fetus is not immunocompetent and cannot remove antibody-coated red cells.
    **D  False** – Parvovirus infection is the commonest identifiable cause of fetal hydrops.

**7.61    Answers**

    **A  True** – Not indicated in Rh+ women.
    **B  False** – Not indicated after complete spontaneous first trimester miscarriage. Indicated if intervention to evacuate the uterus.
    **C  True** – Should be administered after ectopic pregnancy.
    **D  False** – In unsensitized Rh– women, blood is taken for antibody assay at booking, 28 and 34 weeks.

**7.62    Answers**

    **A  False** – The woman is already sensitized – prophylaxis is not required.
    **B  False** – As the woman is Rh– with an affected fetus, her partner must have been Rh+.
    **C  False** – Current partner is heterozygous; therefore, 50% risk of Rh+ fetus.
    **D  False.**

**7.63    Answers**

    **A  False** – Indirect Coombs' test – red cells of a known type are mixed with serum. The addition of anti-human antibodies causes agglutination if the red cells have bound antibody from the serum. Not specific for Rh disease.
    **B  True.**
    **C  False** – See 7.54C.
    **D  False** – Delivery after 34 weeks may be considered safer than continued intrauterine transfusion, although some centres perform transfusions until 36 weeks' gestation.

**7.64    Answers**

    **A  False** – The placenta removes excess bilirubin and the fetus is not jaundiced.
    **B  True** – Fetal anaemia results in increased fetal erythropoietin concentrations, hepatosplenomegaly due to extramedullary erythropoiesis and congestion and the release of red cell precursors (erythroblasts) into the circulation.
    **C  False** – Maternal–fetal ABO incompatibility reduces the risk of Rhesus alloimmunization – ABO antibodies remove fetal red cells before they have time to initiate Rhesus antibody production.
    **D  True** – Bilirubin is excreted in the urine of affected babies.

**7.65**  **Answers**

**A** **True** – Antenatal anti-D prophylaxis has been shown to reduce the risk of maternal sensitization.

**B** **False** – Intrauterine transfusion should be with packed O Rh– red cells compatible with both the mother and fetus.

**C** **False** – Antigens that commonly cause fetal haemolytic disease include Rhesus antigens D, C, E, c, e and Kell antigens.

**D** **False** – First pregnancy may be affected if mother is sensitized following transfusion.

**7.66**  **Answers**

**A** True.
**B** True.
**C** True.
**D** True.

Note: Routine antenatal prophylaxis may not be cost effective or may be unnecessary when the woman (summary of NICE guidelines):

* Has opted to be sterilized after the birth of the baby.
* Is in a stable relationship with the father of the child, and the father is known or found to be RhD–.
* Is certain that she will not have another child after her current pregnancy.
* Is known to be carrying a Rh– fetus.

**7.67**  **Answers**

**A** **False** – Use packed O Rh–red cells compatible with both the mother and fetus.

**B** **False** – See 7.63D.

**C** **False** – Transfuse to supranormal Hb concentration, allowing longer interval between transfusions (2–4 weeks).

**D** **True** – Begin transfusion when haematocrit is below 30%.

**7.68**  **Answers**

**A** True.
**B** False.
**C** False.
**D** False.

**7.69**  **Answers**

**A** False.
**B** False.
**C** True.
**D** False.

## 7.70 Answers

**A** True.
**B** False.
**C** False.
**D** True.

## 7.71 Answers

**A** True.
**B** False.
**C** False.
**D** True.

Note:

- Oligohydramnios: Pool depth devoid of cord/limbs <3 cm (mild), 2 cm (moderate), 1 cm (severe).
- More common in multiple pregnancy.
- Fetal risks: associated with PPROM, IUGR and iatrogenic preterm delivery; pulmonary hypoplasia – mainly dependent on gestational age at PPROM; postural deformities – talipes/Potter facies.
- Causes: PPROM, IUGR, post-maturity, fetal anomaly – renal agenesis/dysplasia, polycystic/multicystic kidney disease, urinary tract obstruction, chromosomal anomaly, fetal infection.

## 7.72 Answers

**A** True – NSAIDs reduce fetal urine output and are recognized treatment.
**B** True.
**C** True – Corticosteroids are beneficial in improving fetal lung maturity.
**D** False – Although diabetes mellitus is a recognized cause of polyhydramnios, the question refers to *idiopathic* polyhydramnios.

## 7.73 Answers

**A** False.
**B** False.
**C** False.
**D** True.

Note: Fetal causes of polyhydramnios:

- GI obstruction – duodenal/oesophageal atresia, diaphragmatic hernia.
- Impaired swallowing – anencephaly, muscular dystrophies.
- Congenital infection – syphilis/hepatitis.
- Chromosomal anomalies.
- Cardiac failure – secondary to anaemia (Rhesus/parvovirus B19/chronic feto-maternal haemorrhage)/chorioangioma.
- Fetal polyuria – TTTS.

**7.74    Answers**
  **A False** – Perinatal mortality rates are 37/1000 (twins), 52/1000 (triplets) and 231/1000 (higher multiples).
  **B False** – Maternal mortality is not significantly increased.
  **C True** – Incidence of monozygotic twins is constant worldwide ~3.5 per 1000.
  **D True** – Dizygotic twins are more common – incidence varies dependent on maternal age (increased with increased maternal age), geographical location (high incidence in Nigeria, low in Japan), assisted conception.

**7.75    Answers**

  **A True** – Monozygotic twins develop from the same embryo and are identical.
  **B True** – Monochorionic twins are always identical. Two-thirds of monozygotic twins are monochorionic.
  **C True** – Dichorionic twins may be identical.
  **D False** – Discordant growth is diagnosed when EFW differ by >20%.

**7.76    Answers**

  **A True.**
  **B True.**
  **C True** – C/S if first twin is breech but vaginal delivery permissible for second twin in a breech presentation, although the optimal mode of delivery remains uncertain.
  **D False.**

**7.77    Answers**

  **A False** – Maternal risks include increased risk of PPH, operative delivery, excessive pregnancy symptoms, hypertensive disorders, gestational diabetes.
  **B False.**
  **C False** – There is no place for intermittent auscultation in the intrapartum management of twins.
  **D False** – Abnormal fetal heart pattern in twin 2 should be managed by C/S if vaginal delivery is not immediately possible.

**7.78    Answers**

  **A False** – Routine prophylactic use of corticosteroids is not recommended.
  **B False** – Tocolytics are not contraindicated but should be used with caution.
  **C False** – Congenital anomalies are more common but aneuploidies are not.
  **D False.**

## 7.79 Answers

**A** **False.**

**B** **False** – Not associated with chromosomal anomalies. Karyotype not indicated unless other anomalies present (<10% associated with other structural anomalies).

**C** **False** – Aim for vaginal delivery in a tertiary centre in co-ordination with neonatal team.

**D** **True** – Increased risk of unexplained intrauterine death near term – close monitoring required.

Note:

- Gastroschisis is a para-umbilical defect, usually right sided. Free floating loops of bowel within amniotic cavity.
- ~1:3000 deliveries. Incidence appears to be increasing. Exomphalos is persistence of physiological herniation.
- Associated with raised MSAFP, polyhydramnios and IUGR.

## 7.80 Answers

**A** **False** – Gut is covered by membrane with cord inserted upon it.

**B** **True** – Persistence of the herniation of the gut into the extra-embryonic part of the umbilical cord, which is usually present between 6th and 14th week of intrauterine life.

**C** **True** – Raised MSAFP. (Amniotic fluid electrophoresis shows faint acetylcholinesterase band and dense pseudo-cholinesterase band [opposite to NTD]).

**D** **True** – 60–80% associated with other anomalies, polyhydramnios, IUGR or chromosomal anomalies (~15%).

## 7.81 Answers

**A** **True.**

**B** **False** – Karyotype not indicated for isolated gastroschisis.

**C** **True.**

**D** **True.**

Note: Fetal karyotype indicated in:

- Duodenal atresia/atrioventricular septal defect – associated with Down.
- Exomphalos – 15% associated with chromosomal anomaly.
- Cystic hygroma, cleft lip and congenital diaphragmatic hernia.

## 7.82 Answers

**A** True.
**B** False.
**C** True.
**D** False.

Note:

- Immune fetal hydrops – associated with anti-D Rhesus antibodies, antibodies to K (Kell system), antibodies to Fya (Duffy system).
- Non-immune hydrops. Idiopathic (30%). Causes:
  1. Infections: parvovirus B19, syphilis, CMV, toxoplasmosis, herpes simplex, leptospirosis, Chagas disease.
  2. Anaemia: secondary to fetal infection, homozygous alpha-thalassaemia, chronic feto-maternal haemorrhage, twin-to-twin transfusion.
  3. Chromosomal anomalies: trisomies, Turner's, triploidy.
  4. Structural anomalies: cardiac – severe congenital heart disease/premature closure of ductus arteriosus/arrhythmias/myocarditis.
  5. Pulmonary – CAML/pulmonary hypoplasia/diaphragmatic hernia.
  6. Renal anomalies.
  7. Anomalies associated with fetal immobility, inborn errors of metabolism, placental chorioangioma.
  8. Maternal disease – diabetes mellitus, pre-eclampsia, severe anaemia/hypoalbuminaemia.

## 7.83 Answers

**A** True.
**B** True.
**C** True.
**D** True.

Note: Fetal hydrops: investigations

- Maternal: FBC, U&E, LFT, urate, blood group + antibodies; Hb electrophoresis (depending on ethnic group); MSAFP; infection screen – TORCH + parvovirus B19 + syphilis + coxsackie; Kleihauer, GTT, lupus anticoagulant + anti-Ro antibodies if bradyarrhythmia.
- Fetal: detailed ultrasound scan – severity of hydrops, anomaly scan with detailed cardiac scan; biophysical assessment; fetal blood sampling – FBC, group, Coombs' test, karyotype, Hb electrophoresis if required + PCR-based infection screen/antibody screen for infection.

## 7.84 Answers

**A** True.
**B** False.
**C** True.
**D** True.

Note: Fetal death in utero is associated with:

- Placental: IUGR, placental abruption, twin-to-twin transfusion syndrome, placental infarction, feto-maternal haemorrhage, trauma including ECV.
- Maternal systemic illness: diabetes mellitus, hypertensive disorders, maternal infections causing septicaemia and hypotension, thrombophilias such as SLE and antiphospholipid antibody syndrome.
- Fetal causes: malformations, chromosomal anomalies, viral and bacterial infections – parvovirus, TORCH, listeriosis, immune haemolytic disease, cord accidents, fetal metabolic disorders.

**7.85 Answers**

    **A** **False** – Normal score = 10. Score of 8 is abnormal especially if associated with oligohydramnios.

    **B** **True** – Fall in BPP score is associated with increased perinatal mortality and morbidity.

    **C** **False.**

    **D** **False** – BPP useful at all gestational ages, although nearer term concerns about fetal well-being are managed by delivery.

Note: Biophysical profile:

- Forms part of comprehensive fetal assessment.
- Includes: fetal breathing movements, gross body/limb movements, fetal tone and posture, fetal heart rate reactivity (CTG), amniotic fluid volume – detects fetal distress before significant brain injury.

**7.86 Answers**

    **A** **False.**

    **B** **True.**

    **C** **True** – Previous preterm labour is the most important predictive risk factor.

    **D** **True.**

**7.87 Answers**

    **A** **True.**

    **B** **True.**

    **C** **True.**

    **D** **True** – Antibiotic treatment in women with spontaneous preterm labour with intact membranes is not associated with improved pregnancy outcome (ORACLE trial).

**7.88 Answers**

    **A** **True.**

    **B** **True.**

    **C** **False.**

    **D** **True** – See 7.86C.

**7.89 Answers**

A **False.**
B **True.**
C **True.**
D **False.**

Note: Risk factors for preterm labour:

- Previous preterm labour.
- Multiple pregnancy, polyhydramnios, cervical incompetence.
- Fetal anomalies.
- Bleeding in pregnancy – threatened miscarriage/APH.
- Infection – UTI in particular.
- Low socioeconomic status, black ethinc group, alcohol and drug abuse, extremes of maternal age, smoking, manual labour/working long hours, pregnancies resulting from assisted conception.
- Cone biopsy, but not LLETZ or cryotherapy, is associated with cervical incompetence and preterm delivery.

**7.90 Answers**

A **True** – $MgSO_4$ is commonly used in USA.
B **True.**
C **True.**
D **False.**

**7.91 Answers**

A **True** – Beta-agonists – ritodrine is the most commonly used beta-agonist, but others include salbutamol and terbutaline. Use limited by side effects. Nitric oxide donors may be as effective as ritodrine and have fewer side effects.
B **True.**
C **False.**
D **False.**

**7.92 Answers**

A **True** – Ethanol is an effective tocolytic but is no longer used clinically.
B **True** – Nimesulide is a specific COX II inhibitor and may therefore be an effective tocolytic without adverse effects on fetal ductal flow or renal function. Non-selective COX inhibitors like indomethacin are also effective. Sulindac has fewer fetal side effects (amniotic fluid and ductus closure).
C **True** – Calcium channel blocker. Nifedipine is commonly used but is not licensed in the UK.
D **True** – Atosiban is an oxytocin antagonist – newer drug. Similar efficacy to ritodrine with fewer side effects.

**7.93** **Answers**

**A** False.

**B** False – Preterm delivery rates are not reduced significantly by tocolysis.

**C** False – Tocolytics are associated with a delay in delivery of 24–48 hours. This on its own is not associated with a significant reduction in perinatal mortality or morbidity. The administration of corticosteroids, however, is associated with a significant reduction in perinatal mortality and morbidity.

**D** False.

**7.94** **Answers**

**A** False.

**B** False.

**C** False.

**D** True – Antenatal corticosteroids significantly reduce the risk of RDS, neonatal death and intraventricular haemorrhage, and reduce cost and duration of neonatal intensive care.

Note:

- RDS affects 40–50% of babies born before 32 weeks' gestation.
- Corticosteroids benefit all major groups of premature babies irrespective of race or gender.
- Numbers needed to treat increases after 34 weeks (5 at <31 weeks, 94 at > 34 weeks).
- RCOG recommends treatment between 24 and 34 weeks. Corticosteroids should be considered between 35 and 36 weeks.
- Optimal treatment to delivery interval is 24 hours to 7 days. Trend towards benefit in babies delivered outside this period.
- No known maternal/fetal side effects.

**7.95** **Answers**

**A** True – Severe maternal systemic infections such as TB and pyelonephritis are contraindications to corticosteroids.

**B** False.

**C** True – Corticosteroids should not be administered if delivery is imminent.

**D** False – Prednisolone does not cross the placenta in sufficient quantities and beta-methasone (or other suitable corticosteroid) should still be administered to women on prednisolone.

**7.96** **Answers**

**A** True.

**B** False.

**C** False.

**D** False

Note: See 7.94.

### 7.97 Answers

**A** **False** – Although the WHO considers fetal viability at 20 weeks, corticosteroids are not recommended at this gestation.

**B** **False** – Tocolytics are not of value.

**C** **True** – The aetiology of PPROM is unknown in the majority of cases but infection is the most likely identifiable cause.

**D** **False** – The terminal alveoli develop at about 22–24 weeks and require amniotic fluid pressure. PPROM at 20 weeks carries a risk of pulmonary hypoplasia.

### 7.98 Answers

**A** **False** – At 20 weeks, management should be expectant after counselling by the obstetrician and neonatologist.

**B** **False.**

**C** **True** – TOP should be recommended if there is evidence of sepsis.

**D** **True** – Complications include miscarriage, preterm delivery, infection, pulmonary hypoplasia and postural deformities.

### 7.99 Answers

**A** **True** – Perinatal outcome is improved by prophylactic erythromycin (ORACLE trial).

**B** **True** – Co-amoxiclav is associated with improved perinatal outcome and with increased risk of neonatal necrotizing enterocolitis.

**C** **True** – Factors causing PPROM include bacterial products and intrinsic weakness in the fetal membranes.

**D** **False** – Cervical cerclage is contraindicated in the presence of ruptured membranes. If a suture is in situ, it should be removed if membranes rupture.

### 7.100 Answers

**A** **True** – Corticosteroids are recommended – improve perinatal outcome.

**B** **True** – Tocolytics are recommended – improve perinatal outcome.

**C** **False** – Erythromycin is not associated with improved outcome in threatened preterm labour with intact membranes.

**D** **False** – Fetal heart would be normal in mild concealed abruption.

### 7.101 Answers

**A** **True** – Constant abdominal pain (especially with uterine tenderness) is suggestive of placental abruption.

**B** **False** – Ultrasound is not a sensitive technique in the detection of placental abruption – diagnosis should be clinical.

**C** **False.**

**D** **True** – A positive Kleihauer test would confirm feto-maternal haemorrhage. This test is, however, not useful in the acute management of placental abruption.

## 7.102 Answers

    **A** **False** – Fibronectin is produced by the chorion.
    **B** **True.**
    **C** **False** – Low sensitivity in predicting delivery within 10 days or before 34 weeks, even in symptomatic women.
    **D** **False** – High negative predictive value (>95%) in asymptomatic women – negative test means the woman is unlikely to deliver in the next 10–14 days.

Note:
- Present in cervico-vaginal secretions in the first and early second trimester of normal pregnancy.

## 7.103 Answers

    **A** **False** – Side effects of nifedipine: headache, flushing, tachycardia, palpitations, hypotension, constipation or diarrhoea, eye pain, visual disturbance.
    **B** **False** – Side effects of ritodrine: flushing, nausea, vomiting, tachycardia, palpitations, hypotension, pulmonary oedema, *hypo*kalaemia, SOB, arrhythmias.
    **C** **True** – Indomethacin can impair fetal renal function causing oligohydramnios. Premature closure of the ductus arteriosus.
    **D** **True** – Side effects of MgSO4: nausea and vomiting, thirst, hypotension, respiratory depression, drowsiness, loss of deep tendon reflexes, muscle weakness.

## 7.104 Answers

    **A** **False** – See 7.103D.
    **B** **False** – Side effects of atosiban: nausea and vomiting, tachycardia, hypotension, headache, hot flushes, hyperglycaemia.
    **C** **True** – See 7.103B.
    **D** **True** – See 7.103A.

### 7.105 Answers

**A** **False** – Not contraindicated in multiple pregnancy, although the evidence that they are effective is weaker than for singleton pregnancies, and the most effective dose is uncertain.

**B** **True** – IDDM is a relative contraindication to the use of corticosteroids, which worsen glycaemic control and may be particularly problematical if used with beta-adrenergic tocolytics.

**C** **False** – PPROM in the absence of infection is not a contraindication to corticosteroids. The risk of infection is not increased.

**D** **True** – Delivery should be considered if chorioamnionitis is suspected. Delay to administer steroids (>24 h) may worsen outcome.

### 7.106 Answers

**A** **False** – Up to 18% of preterm breech infants have a congenital anomaly compared to 5% at term and ~2.5% with term cephalic presentation. Incidence varies with gestational age – 14% at 29–32 weeks, 2–4% at term.

**B** **False** – Female:male ratio = 9:1. First borns are at increased risk.

**C** **True.**

**D** **True** – Risk increased with breech presentation – highest risk with frank breech. Mode of delivery in breech presentation does not influence risk.

### 7.107 Answers

**A** **False** – Early preterm ECV (before 36 weeks' gestation) does not significantly alter the risk of breech presentation at term, caesarean section or perinatal outcome.

**B** **True** – Recent USS is a prerequisite for ECV – normal fetus, presentation and normal liquor volume; as are a reactive CTG, informed consent, facilities to perform C/S.

**C** **True** – Contraindications are: multiple pregnancy, APH, placenta previa, ruptured membranes, fetal anomaly, C/S required for other indication. Relative contraindications include: previous C/S, IUGR, pre-eclampsia, obesity, fetal macrosomia, Rhesus disease.

**D** **False** – Tocolytics (ritodrine) improve the success rate of ECV in nullips (25–43%) but not in multips.

### 7.108 Answers

**A** **False** – Success rate for ECV higher in trials undertaken in black African women compared to Caucasians – tendency to late engagement of the presenting part in black Africans.

**B** **False** – Optimal mode of delivery for preterm breech remains uncertain.

**C** **True** – Associated with increased perinatal mortality even after C/S and correction for gestational age, congenital defects and birth weight.

**D** **False** – 50% of fetuses with hydrocephalus and myelomeningocele present by the breech position.

## 7.109 Answers

**A** **True.**

**B** **False** – Breech fetuses have a *reduced* feto-placental ratio and an *increased* head circumference regardless of mode of delivery.

**C** **True.**

**D** **True.**

Note:

- Breech presentation is associated with: short umbilical cord, abnormal uterine shape, placenta previa and cornual placenta, contracted pelvis, extended legs in the fetus, multiple pregnancy, maternal anticonvulsant use and substance abuse.

**8.1** In women with dysfunctional uterine bleeding:

A There is an increase in endometrial fibrinolytic activity.
B There is a decrease in endometrial prostaglandin $PGE_2$-alpha.
C There is an increase in endometrial prostaglandin $PGF_2$-alpha.
D Aspirin significantly reduces menstrual loss.

**8.2** In a 47-year-old woman with dysfunctional uterine bleeding:

A Combined sequential HRT is effective treatment.
B The low dose combined oral contraceptive pill is contraindicated.
C Tranexamic acid is associated with a significant reduction in menstrual loss.
D The MIRENA intrauterine system is associated with an increased risk of ovarian cysts.

**8.3** A 38-year-old woman complains of regular heavy periods but no other symptoms and no abnormality is detected on examination:

A Endometrial sampling is recommended.
B If she is a smoker, the low dose combined oral contraceptive pill is contraindicated.
C Norethisterone administered for 5–10 days during the luteal phase is effective in reducing menstrual loss.
D Norethisterone administered for 21 days per cycle is effective in reducing menstrual loss.

**8.4** Tranexamic acid:

A Is a prostaglandin synthase inhibitor.
B Reduces menstrual blood loss in women with a copper IUCD.
C Reduces uterine blood loss in women with uterine fibroids.
D Is associated with a lower reduction in menstrual blood loss compared to mefenamic acid.

8.5 Gestrinone:

A Is a 19-nor-testosterone derivative.
B Is an antiandrogen.
C Is an antioestrogen.
D Is an antiprogestogen.


8.6 Endometrial resection/ablation:

A Is associated with an 80% amenorrhoea rate.
B Is associated with a 20% re-operation rate.
C Is not recommended in women who desire amenorrhoea.
D Has resulted in a significant reduction in the number of women undergoing hysterectomy in the UK.


8.7 Endometrial resection/ablation:

A May be associated with hyperkalaemia.
B May be associated with pulmonary oedema.
C May be associated with hypernatraemia.
D Renders the woman infertile and further contraception is unnecessary.


8.8 Endometriosis:

A Is associated with fixed retroversion of the uterus.
B Typically presents with menorrhagia.
C May present with bilateral pelvic masses.
D Is a recognized cause of infertility.


8.9 In a 30-year-old woman complaining of severe dysmenorrhoea and deep dyspareunia:

A Treatment with the combined oral contraceptive pill can be undertaken without a firm diagnosis of endometriosis.
B GnRH agonists are more effective than the combined oral contraceptive pill in relieving endometriosis-associated pain.
C Danazol should be taken from days 2–6 of the cycle.
D Further contraceptive measures are unnecessary once GnRH agonists have been started.

8.10 With respect to the medical management of endometriosis:

A Gestrinone is an oestrogenic antiandrogen.
B Progestogen therapy should be prescribed from days 10–25 of the cycle.
C Progestogen therapy can be continued indefinitely.
D Danazol therapy may be continued indefinitely.

8.11 Danazol:

A Is licensed for the treatment of menorrhagia.
B Can virilize a female fetus.
C Is contraceptive and further contraceptive therapy is unnecessary during treatment.
D Is associated with weight gain.

8.12 The following are recognized side effects of danazol:

A Galactorrhoea.
B Acne.
C Hirsutism.
D De-masculinization of a male fetus.

8.13 The following are recognized side effects of danazol:

A Virilization of a female fetus.
B Reduced breast size.
C Deepening of the voice.
D Hepatocellular carcinoma.

8.14 In a 30-year-old woman with severe endometriosis and infertility:

A IVF has a higher success rate compared to a woman with tubal disease.
B Intrauterine insemination is effective therapy.
C Ovulation induction is effective therapy.
D Ovarian stimulation with intrauterine insemination has been shown to be more effective than no treatment.

8.15 In a 30-year-old woman with severe endometriosis and infertility:

A Treatment with GnRH agonists for 6 months significantly improves spontaneous pregnancy rates.

B Ovarian suppression with danazol for 6 months significantly improves spontaneous pregnancy rates.

C Ovarian suppression with medroxyprogesterone acetate for 6 months is ineffective in improving spontaneous pregnancy rates.

D Ovulation induction is associated with an increased risk of ovarian hyperstimulation compared to women with PCOS.

8.16 Gonadotrophin-releasing hormone analogues:

A Can be administered orally.

B Are associated with a significant reduction in menstrual blood loss.

C May be used to suppress endometrial growth prior to endometrial ablation.

D Suppress ovarian function.

8.17 Anovulation is characteristically associated with:
A Dysmenorrhoea.
B Endometriosis.
C Premenstrual tension.
D Chronic renal failure.

## 8.1 Answers

A **True.**

B **False.**

C **False** – Associated with increased endometrial concentration of vasodilatory prostaglandin $PGE_2$-alpha.

D **False** – Aspirin has not been shown to reduce menstrual blood loss and may in theory increase bleeding.

## 8.2 Answers

A **True** – Sequential HRT is effective treatment for perimenopausal DUB.

B **False** – The COCP is not contraindicated on the basis of age alone.

C **True** – Tranexamic acid, mefenamic acid and the COCP are RCOG recommended first-line treatments in primary/secondary care.

D **True.**

## 8.3 Answers

A **False** – In women under the age of 40 years with menorrhagia, no other symptoms and a normal pelvic examination, no further investigations are required prior to treatment.

B **True** – The COCP is contraindicated in smokers over 35 years.

C **False** – Systemic progestogens are ineffective in the treatment of ovulatory dysfunctional uterine bleeding when low doses are used for 5–10 days in the luteal phase.

D **True** – Norethisterone is effective if given at higher doses (5 mg three times a day) for 3 weeks out of 4.

## 8.4 Answers

A **False** – Tranexamic acid is an antifibrinolytic agent.

B **True** – Effective in reducing menstrual loss associated with IUCD, fibroids and bleeding diathesis.

C **True.**

D **False** – Reduces menstrual loss by ~50% and is more effective than NSAIDs.

Note:

- Not associated with an increased risk of DVT.
- Side effects – nausea/vomiting/diarrhoea; disturbance in colour vision – discontinue therapy.

## 8.5 Answers

**A** True.
**B** False.
**C** True.
**D** True.

Note:
- Gestrinone is administered twice weekly.
- Significantly reduces menstrual loss but not first-line therapy.
- Not licensed for the treatment of menorrhagia.
- Associated with androgenic side effects (milder than danazol) and can virilize female fetus; therefore, barrier contraception is essential.

## 8.6 Answers

**A** **False** – Amenorrhoea rates 20–40%.
**B** **True** – Associated with a re-operation rate of up to 38% at 3 years (10–25% require hysterectomy after 3–4 years).
**C** **True** – Pre-operative counselling and patient selection is vital – women should have heavy menses and should not expect amenorrhoea.
**D** **False.**

Note:
- Endometrial ablative procedures are effective in treating menorrhagia.
- Associated with lower morbidity and quicker recovery compared to hysterectomy, with a significant improvement in Hb and quality of life. Risk of fluid overload.
- Long-term satisfaction rates ~80%.

## 8.7 Answers

**A** **False.**
**B** **True.**
**C** **False** – Fluid retention may cause *hypo*natraemia with pulmonary/cerebral oedema.
**D** **False** – Women need to continue contraception as there is a risk of pregnancy.

## 8.8 Answers

**A** **True** – Clinical findings may include a fixed retroverted uterus and pelvic mass (endometrioma). In most women, pelvic tenderness is the only finding.
**B** **False** – Typically presents with chronic pelvic pain, dysmenorrhoea and deep dyspareunia.
**C** **True.**
**D** **True** – The effect of minimal to mild endometriosis on fertility is controversial. Severe endometriosis with pelvic adhesions is associated with subfertility.

## 8.9 Answers

**A** **True** – In women with symptoms of endometriosis, empirical treatment with the COCP may be undertaken without need for laparoscopy.

**B** **False** – There is no evidence that any medical treatment is superior. Therapies are limited by their side effects.

**C** **False** – Danazol should be taken on a continuous basis.

**D** **False** – GnRH agonists are not licensed contraceptives.

## 8.10 Answers

**A** **False** – See 8.5.

**B** **False** – Progestogens are used on a continuous basis in sufficient dose to induce amenorrhoea – effective in relieving pain.

**C** **False** – Prolonged use may lead to hypo-oestrogenaemia and loss of bone mineral density – limit to 6 months.

**D** **False** – Treatment with danazol should be for up to 6 months.

## 8.11 Answers

**A** **True.**

**B** **True** – Women must be advised to use barrier contraception as danazol can virilize a female fetus if pregnancy occurs.

**C** **False.**

**D** **True** – Weight gain of 2–4 kg with 3-month treatment.

Note:

- Synthetic androgen with antioestrogenic and antiprogestogenic activity.
- Reduces menstrual loss but is associated with androgenic side effects: weight gain, acne, hirsutism, seborrhoea, irritability, musculoskeletal pains, fatigue, hot flushes and breast atrophy.

## 8.12 Answers

**A** False.

**B** True.

**C** True.

**D** False.

## 8.13 Answers

**A** True.

**B** True.

**C** True.

**D** False.

Note: Side effects of danazol:

- Androgenic side effects such as acne, oily skin, breast atrophy, weight gain, hirsutism and vaginal dryness. Voice changes and rarely clitoral hypertrophy may occur.
- Changes in libido (usually increased) due to androgenic effects.
- Skin reactions including rash, photosensitivity and exfoliative dermatitis.

- Androgenic effects may cause virilization of a female fetus.
- Associated with benign hepatic adenomas.
- Associated with benign hepatic adenomas but not carcinoma.

### 8.14 Answers

**A False** – IVF embryo transfer is effective treatment for endometriosis-associated infertility. The effect of endometriosis on the outcome of IVF is controversial, with some studies suggesting lower pregnancy rates.

**B False.**

**C False.**

**D False** – There is *no* place for ovarian hyperstimulation if there is evidence of distortion of tubal anatomy. However, ovarian stimulation with intrauterine insemination is better than no treatment in women with minimal to mild disease.

### 8.15 Answers

**A False** – There is no place for medical treatment in the management of endometriosis-related subfertility.

**B False.**

**C True.**

**D False** – PCOS is associated with an increased risk of OHSS.

### 8.16 Answers

**A False** – GnRH analogues are polypeptides and are not active orally.

**B True** – Result in amenorrhoea but are associated with menopausal symptoms and loss of bone mineral density.

**C True** – May be used over the short-term for intractable menorrhagia or to suppress endometrial growth prior to TCRE or to reduce the size of fibroids prior to myomectomy.

**D True.**

### 8.17 Answers

**A False** – Anovulatory cycles typically do not cause dysmenorrhoea.

**B False** – There is no association between endometriosis and anovulation.

**C False** – PMT shows cyclical symptoms and is not associated with anovulation.

**D True** – Chronic illness, including renal failure, typically results in anovulation.

**9.1** Toxoplasmosis in a pregnant woman:

A Is caused by a Gram-negative bacterium.
B Is usually asymptomatic.
C Usually presents with posterior cervical lymphadenopathy.
D In the first trimester is associated with spontaneous miscarriage.

**9.2** Toxoplasmosis in a pregnant woman:

A A four-fold rise in IgG titres from blood samples 3 weeks apart indicates acute infection.
B Can be contracted from raw meat and cat faeces.
C Spiramycin is ineffective after 20 weeks' gestation.
D Is sensitive to pyrimethamine.

**9.3** With respect to toxoplasmosis in pregnancy:

A The disease can be contracted by eating raw, poorly washed vegetables.
B Hydrocephalus is a recognized complication of fetal infection.
C Hepatitis is a recognized complication of fetal infection.
D The fetus is more severely affected when infection occurs in late pregnancy.

**9.4** With respect to toxoplasmosis in pregnancy:

A When primary infection occurs in pregnancy, the fetus is infected in about 40% of cases.
B Pregnancy re-activates latent disease.
C Spiramycin is more effective than pyrimethamine or sulfadiazine in treating the affected fetus.
D A positive specific antitoxoplasma IgM test in the serum indicates acute infection.

9.5 With respect to toxoplasmosis in pregnancy:

A The incidence of infection in pregnant women in the UK is 2 per 1000 pregnancies.
B About 95% of maternal infections are transmitted to the fetus.
C Spiramycin is used to treat in utero infection.
D Evidence of prior infection is present in over 50% of women of reproductive age in the UK.

9.6 Listeriosis:

A Is caused by a Gram-negative anaerobe.
B Is more common in patients with depressed T-cell-mediated immunity.
C Is most common in the third trimester.
D First trimester infection may result in spontaneous miscarriage.

9.7 Listeriosis:

A Early-onset neonatal disease is caused by horizontal or nosocomial spread.
B Late-onset neonatal disease usually presents with meningitis.
C Maternal cultures are usually positive in late-onset neonatal disease.
D Is treated with ampicillin.

9.8 Cytomegalovirus infection causes:

A Microcephaly.
B IUGR.
C Fetal hydrops.
D Hydrocephalus.

9.9 Cytomegalovirus infection:

A Causes intracranial calcification.
B Can be treated with acyclovir.
C Neonatal infection may occur through breast milk.
D Primary infection occurs in 2% of pregnant women.

**9.10** A baby born to a woman who is hepatitis B surface antigen positive:

A The baby is more likely to be infected in utero than during delivery.

B Hepatitis B immune globulin should be administered to the neonate within 12 hours of delivery.

C The first dose of hepatitis B vaccine should be administered at 1 month.

D The second and third doses of hepatitis B vaccine should be administered at 1 and 6 months.

**9.11** A 35-year-old woman presents with primary genital herpes at 30 weeks' gestation:

A Herpes simplex virus type I is the most likely cause.

B The disease may have resulted from contact with a partner with orolabial herpes.

C The disease can be contracted from an asymptomatic partner.

D Encephalitis and meningitis are recognized complications.

**9.12** A 35-year-old woman presents with primary genital herpes at 30 weeks' gestation:

A Preterm delivery is a known complication.

B Acyclovir is contraindicated.

C Weekly swabs for viral culture are recommended for the rest of the pregnancy.

D There is an absolute indication for caesarean section at 39 weeks' gestation.

**9.13** Rubella infection in pregnancy:

A Occurring at 8 weeks' gestation results in a high rate of fetal infection.

B Occurring at 40 weeks' gestation results in a high rate of fetal infection.

C Occurring at 8 weeks' gestation results in a high proportion of fetuses being affected.

D Occurring at 40 weeks' gestation results in a high proportion of fetuses being affected.

9.14 Rubella infection in pregnancy:

A Is associated with congenital heart defects.
B Is effectively prevented by the MMR vaccine.
C Immunity acquired from vaccination is life-long.
D Termination of pregnancy should be offered if immunization occurs during the first trimester.

9.15 Rubella infection in pregnancy:

A Is the commonest cause of congenital heart defects.
B Has an incubation period of 10–21 days.
C Detection of rubella IgM implies immunity to rubella.
D Following contact, is effectively prevented by rubella immune globulin.

9.16 Rubella infection in pregnancy:

A The presence of rubella IgG in cord blood confirms congenital infection.
B Is caused by a DNA virus.
C Can be treated with intravenous acyclovir.
D Is associated with IUGR.

9.17 Rubella infection in pregnancy:

A Is associated with congenital deafness.
B Is associated with cutaneous scarring in a dermatomal pattern.
C Is associated with a characteristic rash.
D Fetal infection can be diagnosed by cordocentesis.

9.18 Rubella infection in the first trimester is associated with a subsequent increase in the risk of:

A Phocomelia.
B IUGR.
C Oligohydramnios.
D Neonatal purpura.

9.19 Rubella infection in the first trimester is associated with a subsequent increase in the risk of:

A Microcephaly.
B Insulin-dependent diabetes mellitus.
C Intracranial calcification.
D Thyroid disease.

9.20 Congenital rubella:

A Can be prevented by the administration of immunoglobulins to an infected mother during pregnancy.
B Is likely to follow accidental vaccination during the first trimester.
C May result in excretion of the rubella virus for more than 6 months.
D Does not occur following maternal infection in the second trimester.

9.21 Chorioamnionitis:

A Is a recognized cause of preterm labour.
B Does not occur in the absence of maternal pyrexia.
C Can be prevented by the use of prophylactic erythromycin in preterm premature rupture of the membranes.
D Is associated with early amniotomy in labour.

9.22 Chorioamnionitis:

A Is always accompanied by fetal tachycardia.
B At 34 weeks' gestation should prompt delivery by caesarean section.
C Is usually caused by coliforms only.
D Is associated with an increased risk of respiratory distress in preterm neonates.

9.23 Gonococcal infection in pregnancy:

A Is usually symptomatic.
B Pharyngitis is more common than in the non-pregnant.
C Disseminated infection is less common.
D Diagnosis is confirmed by the identification of Gram-positive intracellular diplococci.

9.24 With respect to maternal infection with *Chlamydia trachomatis*:

A Blindness is a recognized complication.
B The majority of infected women are asymptomatic.
C Neonatal pneumonia is a recognized complication.
D In the first trimester is associated with increased risk of miscarriage.

9.25   Chancroid:

A  Is caused by a protozoan.
B  Is sexually transmitted.
C  Is caused by *Treponema pallidum*.
D  Is associated with painful inguinal lymphadenopathy.

9.26   Postpartum endometritis:

A  Is less common after vaginal delivery compared to caesarean section.
B  Is effectively prevented by the use of prophylactic antibiotics at caesarean section.
C  Is a polymicrobial infection.
D  Is associated with antepartum bacterial vaginosis.

9.27   Puerperal pyrexia:

A  May be due to breast engorgement.
B  Secondary to mastitis is usually caused by coliforms.
C  Associated with erythema and breast tenderness should be treated with flucloxacillin.
D  Thromboembolism is a recognized cause.

9.28   With respect to parvovirus B19 infection in pregnancy:

A  Immune hydrops is the most frequent finding in infected fetuses.
B  The infection can be contracted from an infected pet.
C  There is a 25% risk of fetal death in an infected pregnancy.
D  The virus shortens the life-span of red blood cells.

9.29   With respect to parvovirus B19 infection in pregnancy:

A  Erythema infectiosum is the most common clinical presentation.
B  The majority of women presenting with clinical features of parvovirus infection are infectious.
C  Maternal anaemia is a recognized complication in immunocompromised individuals.
D  Infection is an indication for pregnancy termination.

9.30  With respect to parvovirus B19 infection in pregnancy:

    A  Maternal infection carries a vertical transmission rate of ~1%.

    B  The annual seroconversion rate of susceptible primary school employees is greater than that of hospital employees.

    C  Susceptible school teachers should be excluded from the classroom until after 20 weeks' gestation to reduce the risk of infection.

    D  Maternal serum AFP is increased in affected pregnancies.

9.31  With respect to parvovirus B19 infection in pregnancy:

    A  Placental immunohistochemistry is the best investigation to confirm fetal infection.

    B  In school outbreaks, ~20% of susceptible staff will develop serological evidence of infection.

    C  A high fetal reticulocyte count is a poor prognostic sign.

    D  The virus is a typical orphan virus.

9.32  Parvovirus B19 causes aplastic anaemia in adults in the following circumstances:

    A  Pregnancy.

    B  Sickle cell disease.

    C  Thalassaemia.

    D  Pyruvate kinase deficiency.

9.33  The following are typical features of parvovirus B19 infection:

    A  The disease is highly infectious when the rash erupts.

    B  Infection in the first trimester poses the highest risk to the fetus.

    C  Susceptible primary school teachers are at higher risk of infection than susceptible hospital workers.

    D  10% of susceptible adults become infected every year.

9.34  The following are typical features of parvovirus B19 infection:

    A  Detection of viral DNA in maternal serum by PCR is the best way of diagnosing maternal infection in pregnancy.

    B  Detection of viral DNA in fetal tissue is the most sensitive way of detecting fetal infection.

    C  Acyclovir is recognized treatment for maternal infection in pregnancy.

    D  The virus has a predilection for rapidly dividing cells.

**9.35** A 30-year-old woman has been found to be HIV positive on routine screening at 14 weeks' gestation:

A The woman should be encouraged to inform her sexual partner of the diagnosis.

B The woman's HIV status may be disclosed to a sexual partner if the woman cannot be persuaded to do so herself.

C The woman's diagnosis may be disclosed to her next of kin if she cannot be persuaded to do so herself.

D All healthcare professionals caring for the woman should be made aware of the diagnosis.

**9.36** With respect to the mode of delivery in HIV-positive women:

A Elective caesarean section significantly reduces the risk of vertical transmission in women on HAART with undetectable viral loads.

B Caesarean section should be recommended if the membranes have been ruptured for more than 4 hours.

C Clamping of the cord should be delayed.

D If the woman is taking HAART, the risk of vertical transmission is doubled if the membranes are ruptured for >4 hours before delivery.

**9.37** With respect to the mode of delivery in HIV-positive women:

A Elective C/S should be recommended in women not taking HAART.

B In women not taking HAART, i.v. zidovudine should be commenced at least 4 hours before elective C/S.

C In women not taking HAART, there is a 2% increase in the risk of vertical transmission for every hour of ruptured membranes up to 24 hours.

D The baby should be bathed immediately after delivery.

**9.38** With respect to antiretroviral therapy for HIV-positive pregnant women:

A Women with advanced HIV disease should receive HAART during the first trimester.

B HAART should be commenced if the CD4 count is <200–350/L.

C In women who conceive while taking HAART, treatment should be discontinued and re-introduced after the first trimester.

D Zidovudine is the only antiretroviral agent specifically indicated for use during the first trimester.

**9.39** With respect to antiretroviral therapy for HIV-positive pregnant women:

  A Women who do not require antiretroviral therapy for their own health should commence treatment at 28–32 weeks' gestation to reduce the risk of vertical transmission.
  B Women who present with HIV disease late in pregnancy should be treated with single agent zidovudine only.
  C Optimal use of HAART should suppress viral load to <50 copies/ml.
  D Metabolic alkalosis is a recognized complication of HAART regimens.

**9.40** The following investigations are recommended to monitor for drug toxicity in HIV-positive pregnant women taking HAART:

  A FBC.
  B U&E.
  C Serum lactate.
  D Liver function tests.

**9.41** The following investigations are recommended to monitor for drug toxicity in HIV-positive pregnant women taking HAART:

  A Serum glucose.
  B CRP.
  C CD4 count.
  D Echocardiography in each trimester.

**9.42** The following are suggestive of lactic acidosis in a pregnant HIV-positive woman receiving HAART:

  A Proteinuria.
  B Nausea and vomiting.
  C Fever.
  D Breathlessness.

**9.43** The following are associated with an increased risk of vertical transmission of HIV:

  A Advanced maternal disease.
  B High antenatal CD4 count.
  C High maternal viral load.
  D Chorioamnionitis.

9.44 With respect to HIV disease in pregnancy:

    A CD4 count falls during pregnancy and returns to pre-pregnancy levels after delivery.

    B Pregnancy is associated with more rapid progression of HIV disease.

    C Vertical transmission does not occur when the maternal viral load is <1000 copies/ml.

    D 20% of vertical transmission occurs during the first trimester.

9.45 With respect to vaccination:

    A Rabies vaccine is safe for use in pregnancy.

    B Tetanus vaccination carries no risk of fetal infection.

    C If vaccination against polio is required during pregnancy, the Sabin strain should be used.

    D Varicella zoster immune globulin should be administered to the term neonate of a mother who had shingles in the second trimester.

9.46 Eye damage is a recognized consequence of fetal infection with the following organisms:

    A *Treponema pallidum.*

    B *Toxoplasma gondii.*

    C Epstein–Barr virus.

    D Cytomegalovirus.

9.47 The following maternal infections may be transmitted to the neonate as a result of vaginal delivery:

    A HIV virus.

    B HPV virus.

    C *Listeria monocytogenes.*

    D *Falciparum malaria.*

# Answers

## 9.1 Answers

**A** **False** – *Toxoplasma gondii* is obligate intracellular protozoan.

**B** **True** – Human infection is usually asymptomatic/produces glandular fever-like illness.

**C** **True** – Lymphadenopathy involving the posterior cervical chain is the commonest clinical manifestaton.

**D** **True** – Fetal risks include spontaneous first trimester miscarriage, chorioretinitis, IUGR, microcephaly, hydrocephalus, intracranial calcification, learning disability, hepatosplenomegaly.

## 9.2 Answers

**A** **True** – Serology is commonly used for diagnosis but is potentially confusing. An initial positive IgM serology does not necessarily imply current infection. Acute infection confirmed by finding either a four-fold rise in IgG titres in blood drawn 3 weeks apart or high IgM titres (>1:256).

**B** **True** – Infection occurs through ingestion of contaminated food, including vegetable or infected meat.

**C** **False** – Spiramycin therapy to infected mothers – 60% reduction in the risk of fetal infection.

**D** **True** – Pyramethamine + sulfonamide + folinic acid if fetal infection; helps arrest progression of fetal disease.

Note:
- Infected neonates require treatment for the first year of life.
- Risk of fetal infection increases while severity of affection decreases with increasing gestation age.

## 9.3 Answers

**A** **True** – See 9.2B.
**B** **True** – See 9.1D.
**C** **True**.
**D** **False**.

## 9.4 Answers

**A** **True**.
**B** **False**.
**C** **False** – See 9.2D.
**D** **False** – An initial positive IgM serology does not necessarily imply current infection.

Note:
- Overall, 60% of fetuses are born without obvious damage, 10% have chorioretinitis only and 20–30% have multiple anomalies typical of the TORCH syndrome – hydrocephalus, chorioretinitis, intracranial calcification, jaundice, microcephaly, anaemia.

## 9.5    Answers

**A  True** – About 14% of women of reproductive age are immune to toxoplasmosis and about 30% of 30-year-olds are immune. About 1:500 women become infected during pregnancy.

**B  False** – Primary infection in first trimester ~17% of fetuses affected; 25% affected in second and 65% in third trimester. However, with advancing gestation, the severity of fetal damage lessens.

**C  False** – Pyramethamine + sulfadiazine + folinic acid if fetal infection.

**D  False.**

## 9.6    Answers

**A  False** – *Listeria monocytogenes* is a Gram-positive, beta-haemolytic facultative anaerobe.

**B  True** – T-cell immunity is important in the modulation of *L. monocytogenes* infection.

**C  True.**

**D  True** – May cause chorioamnionitis and septic miscarriage or fetal death in utero.

## 9.7    Answers

**A  False** – Early-onset neonatal disease is most common after acute febrile illness in the mother.

**B  True** – Late-onset neonatal disease occurs in term neonates after uncomplicated pregnancy and typically presents with meningitis.

**C  False** – Horizontally acquired and maternal cultures are usually negative.

**D  True** – Commence antibiotics once infection is suspected – sensitive to ampicillin/penicillin. Aminoglycosides are also effective and are usually given in addition to penicillin.

Note:
- Neonate is symptomatic at birth or within a few days of life.
- Associated with disseminated granulomas (granulomatosis infantisepticum) involving liver, placenta and other solid organs, septic shock and respiratory distress.

## 9.8    Answers

**A  True.**

**B  True.**

**C  True.**

**D  True.**

Note: Fetal risks with CMV:
- Commonest cause of congenital sensorineural deafness.
- Hepatosplenomegaly, IUGR.
- Microcephaly, learning disability.
- Thrombocytopenia, jaundice.
- Haemolytic anaemia and hydrops.

## 9.9 Answers

**A** True.

**B** False.

**C** True – Fetus can be infected by transplacental passage of virus or neonate infected by exposure to virus from birth canal/breast milk/exposure to other babies in nursery.

**D** True – Primary infection occurs in ~2% of pregnant women (40–50% are susceptible).

Note:

- DNA virus. Commonest congenital viral infection in pregnancy.
- Causes self-limiting febrile illness in immunocompetent individuals.
- Causes severe illness in immunocompromised, including pneumonia and hepatitis.
- Fetal infection occurs with primary as well as re-activated infection.
- Can be isolated from ~1% of all neonates.

## 9.10 Answers

**A** False – Only 5% of fetuses are infected in utero as a result of transplacental haemorrhage. The rest are infected at birth from maternal blood and body fluids.

**B** True – Neonate should receive Hep B immune globulin within 12 h of delivery.

**C** False – Neonate should receive first dose of Hep B vaccine within 7 days.

**D** True – The second and third doses of Hep B vaccine should be administered at 1 and 6 months and tested for Hep B surface antigen at 12–15 months.

## 9.11 Answers

**A** False – Herpes simplex type I typically causes oro-labial lesions while type II typically causes genital herpes. However, both types can cause genital herpes.

**B** True – Genital herpes can arise following orogenital contact.

**C** True.

**D** True.

Note:

- In most pregnancies complicated by neonatal herpes, the woman is asymptomatic.

## 9.12 Answers

**A** True – Primary infection may be severe enough to cause systemic illness, fever and preterm labour.

**B** False – Acyclovir is not contraindicated in pregnancy.

**C** False – Repeated swabs for viral culture are not effective in reducing the risk of vertical transmission and should not be undertaken.

**D** False – Elective C/S is indicated only for women who present with primary infection at the time of delivery or within 6 weeks of the expected date of delivery or onset of preterm labour.

## 9.13 Answers

**A** **True** – The risk of fetal infection increases in the third trimester and after 36 weeks almost all fetuses will be infected.

**B** **True.**

**C** **True** – Risk of the fetus being affected falls with increasing gestation: >90% in the first trimester with no fetuses being affected after 20 weeks.

**D** **False.**

## 9.14 Answers

**A** **True** – Heart defects include patent ductus arteriosus, pulmonary valvular and artery stenosis, coarctation of the aorta, VSD and ASD.

**B** **True.**

**C** **False** – Vaccination results in long-term (not life-long) immunity in 95% of those vaccinated.

**D** **False** – No evidence that immunization in the first trimester is associated with congenital rubella syndrome; therefore TOP is not indicated.

## 9.15 Answers

**A** **False** – The majority of congenital heart defects are sporadic/polygeneic and are not related to rubella infection.

**B** **True** – Incubation period 2–3 weeks.

**C** **False** – Detection of IgG with high titres indicates immunity.

**D** **False** – Rubella immune globulin is not used to prevent infection after contact.

## 9.16 Answers

**A** **False** – IgM in cord blood would indicate congenital infection.

**B** **False** – Rubella is a DNA virus.

**C** **False** – No antiviral treatment available.

**D** **True** – Consequences of congenital infection include effects on eyes, ears and heart, and IUGR.

## 9.17 Answers

**A** **True** – See 9.19.

**B** **False** – Cutaneous scarring occurs with varicella.

**C** **False** – Rash is not diagnostic.

**D** **True** – Fetal infection may be diagnosed by fetal blood sampling and PCR although this is rarely necessary.

## 9.18 Answers

**A** **False** – Phocomelia (Greek for seal-limb) – short or absent long bones with flipper-like appearance of hands/feet is classically due to thalidomide.

**B** **True.**

**C** **True.**

**D** **True.**

**9.19 Answers**

**A** True.
**B** True.
**C** False.
**D** True.

Note: Rubella infection in the first trimester is associated with:

- Eyes – cataract, retinopathy, glaucoma and micro-ophthalmia.
- Heart – patent ductus arteriosus, pulmonary valvular and artery stenosis, coarctation of the aorta, VSD and ASD.
- Ear – bilateral and progressive hearing loss.
- IUGR and oligohydramnios.
- Neonatal hepatosplenomegaly, purpura, jaundice, meningoencephalitis and thrombocytopenia.
- Increased risk of diabetes mellitus, thyroid disease and rarely growth hormone deficiency in later life.

**9.20 Answers**

**A** False.
**B** False – No case of congenital rubella syndrome as a result of immunization has been documented.
**C** True – Fetal viraemia continues throughout pregnancy and the infant may continue to excrete virus for up to a year.
**D** False – Risk of fetal infection >90% in the first trimester; 25% in early second trimester.

**9.21 Answers**

**A** True.
**B** False – Clinical presentation is characterized by maternal fever, tachycardia, uterine tenderness, fetal tachycardia ± offensive vaginal loss – this complicates 1–2% of all deliveries. Signs and symptoms are non-specific and chorioamnionitis can occur in the absence of maternal pyrexia.
**C** True – In women with PPROM, prophylactic erythromycin is associated with a reduction in the risk of intrauterine infection (ORACLE trial).
**D** False – Early amniotomy in labour does not increase the risk of chorioamnionitis.

Note:

- Histological chorioamnionitis occurs in ~5% of term deliveries and 50% of preterm deliveries.

## 9.22 Answers

**A** **False** – Clinical manifestations such as maternal pyrexia and tachycardia, uterine tenderness and fetal tachycardia are non-specific and are not always present.

**B** **False** – Mode of delivery is dependent on fetal condition and prompt antibiotic therapy with vaginal delivery is usually possible at 34 weeks' gestation.

**C** **False** – Microbes frequently isolated include Group B strep, coliforms, enterococcus, anaerobes, mycoplasma.

**D** **True** – Associated with increased risk of RDS, intraventricular haemorrhage, clinical neonatal sepsis and 3–4-fold increase in perinatal mortality.

## 9.23 Answers

**A** **False** – Usually asymptomatic cervicitis.

**B** **True** – Pharyngitis more common in pregnancy probably as a result of altered sexual practices.

**C** **False** – Disseminated gonococcal infection is more common in pregnancy.

**D** **False** – Confirmed by identification of Gram-negative intracellular diplococcus.

## 9.24 Answers

**A** **True** – Serotypes A,B and C cause endemic trachoma, which is the leading cause of blindness worldwide.

**B** **True** – The majority of infected pregnant women have asymptomatic cervicitis.

**C** **True** – Neonatal complications include conjunctivitis and pneumonia.

**D** **False** – Not associated with increased risk of miscarriage. Recently acquired infection may be associated with increased risk of PPROM and preterm delivery.

## 9.25 Answers

**A** **False** – Caused by *Haemophilus ducreyi*, a Gram-negative bacillus.

**B** **True** – Sexually transmitted, more common in males.

**C** **False** – See A.

**D** **True** – Painful inguinal lymphadenopathy occurs in 50% and may lead to abscess formation.

Note:
- Incubation period 4–7 days.
- Presents with genital ulceration, typically painful in men and painless in females.
- In pregnancy, can be treated with azithromycin, erythromycin or ceftriaxone.

**9.26 Answers**

  **A** **True** – Most common serious complication of the puerperium – more common after C/S compared to vaginal delivery. Exteriorizing the uterus and MROP at C/S may increase the risk.

  **B** **True** – Risk is significantly reduced by the use of prophylactic antibiotics during C/S. Continued antibiotic therapy for over 12 hours post-partum is of no additional benefit.

  **C** **True.**

  **D** **True** – Risk factors include chorioamnionitis, C/S, lower socioeconomic status, colonization with Group B strep, *Gardnerella*, *Chlamydia*, *Mycoplasma*; pre-existing bacterial vaginosis and extremes of maternal age.

**9.27 Answers**

  **A** **True.**

  **B** **False** – Mastitis may occur in the absence of bacterial infection.

  **C** **True** – Flucloxacillin is the antibiotic of choice as *Staph. aureus* is the most likely cause.

  **D** **True.**

Note:
- Pyrexia over 38°C on two occasions after the first 24 hours postpartum.
- Causes of puerperal pyrexia include endometritis, breast engorgement, mastitis, VTE, perineal abscess, haematoma, thrombophlebitis, wound infections, UTI, chest infection.

**9.28 Answers**

  **A** **False** – *Non-immune* fetal hydrops is the most frequent pathological finding in infected fetuses.

  **B** **False** – Not contracted from animals.

  **C** **False** – Fetal loss rate 9%, highest risk in the second trimester.

  **D** **True** – Replicate in, inhibit colony formation and cause lysis of human erythroid progenitor cells.

**9.29 Answers**

  **A** **False** – Pregnant women present with rash/arthralgia.

  **B** **False** – Rash does not occur until 17–18 days after infection and about 5 days after the disappearance of virus from serum and respiratory droplets. Patients presenting with the clinical infection are no longer infectious.

  **C** **True** – Chronic anaemia may occur in immunocompromised individuals.

  **D** **False** – Vertical transmission rate ~30%. Infection is not an indication for termination of pregnancy.

## 9.30 Answers

**A** **False** – Vertical transmission rate ~30%.
**B** **True** – Annual seroconversion rate among susceptible primary school employees is 5.2% compared to 2.4% in hospital staff.
**C** **False.**
**D** **True** – Elevated maternal serum AFP may be a marker of fetal parvovirus B19 infection.

## 9.31 Answers

**A** **False** – PCR is most sensitive way of confirming fetal infection.
**B** **True** – Transmissibility: 50–90% among susceptible household contacts, 20–30% among susceptible staff in schools during outbreaks.
**C** **False** – Fetal reticulocytosis (>20%) is a good prognostic sign and indicates that fetal Hb has probably reached its nadir and spontaneous recovery is likely to occur (34% of cases).
**D** **False** – DNA virus with single-stranded DNA genome.

## 9.32 Answers

**A** **False.**
**B** **True.**
**C** **True.**
**D** **True.**

Note:

- Parvovirus B19 causes transient aplastic crisis in sickle cell disease and other hereditary anaemias, including spherocytosis, thalassaemia, pyruvate kinase deficiency and autoimmune haemolytic anaemia.

## 9.33 Answers

**A** **False** – See 9.29B.
**B** **False.**
**C** **True** – See 9.30B.
**D** **False.**

## 9.34 Answers

**A** **False** – Clinical diagnosis unreliable. Demonstrate specific IgM or seroconversion in paired sera.
**B** **True** – PCR-based testing of fetal blood sample is the most sensitive way of confirming fetal infection.
**C** **False** – Maternal treatment – symptomatic. Fetal – treat hydrops.
**D** **True** – Virus replicates spontaneously only in dividing cells in the S phase of mitosis and has a predilection for rapidly dividing cells.

**9.35 Answers**

- **A** **True** – The woman should be encouraged to inform her sexual partner.
- **B** **True** – It must *not* be assumed that the woman's partner or family are aware of her diagnosis. The woman's HIV status may be disclosed to a known sexual partner to protect him when the woman has not informed him and cannot be persuaded to do so. The woman must be told of such disclosure.
- **C** **False.**
- **D** **True** – All professionals caring for the woman should be aware of the diagnosis and plan of management – she should, however, be re-assured that confidentiality will be respected.

**9.36 Answers**

- **A** **False** – In women taking HAART with undetectable viral load, the value of C/S remains uncertain.
- **B** **False.**
- **C** **False** – Cord should be clamped as early as possible after delivery.
- **D** **False** – Ruptured membranes for >4 hours is associated with double the risk of vertical transmission in women not taking HAART, with a 2% increase in risk for every hour of ruptured membranes up to 24 hours.

**9.37 Answers**

- **A** **True** – In HIV-positive women not taking HAART during pregnancy and those with detectable viral load, delivery by elective C/S (after 38 weeks) reduces the risk of vertical transmission.
- **B** **True** – Start zidovudine infusion 4 h before C/S and continue until cord clamped.
- **C** **True** – See 9.36D.
- **D** **True** – Baby should be bathed immediately after birth.

**9.38 Answers**

- **A** **False** – Women with advanced HIV disease should receive HAART started after the first trimester and continued after delivery.
- **B** **False** – HAART recommended for use in pregnancy (usually at CD4 count of 200–350 *million/L*).
- **C** **False** – Women who conceive while taking HAART should continue treatment if viral load is suppressed. If viral load is not suppressed, therapy should be changed after the first trimester.
- **D** **False** – Zidovudine is specifically indicated for use in pregnancy (except the first trimester) for the prevention of vertical transmission.

## 9.39 Answers

**A** **True** – Women who do not require antiretroviral therapy for their own health but require treatment to prevent vertical transmission from ~28 weeks.

**B** **False** – Women who present with HIV late in pregnancy or in labour should be treated with HAART regimen including zidovudine.

**C** **True** – Optimal use of HAART should suppress viral load to undetectable levels (<50 copies/ml).

**D** **False** – Lactic acidosis is a recognized complication of some HAART regimens.

## 9.40 Answers

**A** True.
**B** True.
**C** True.
**D** True.

## 9.41 Answers

**A** True.
**B** False.
**C** False.
**D** False.

Note:
• Women taking antiretroviral agents should be monitored for drug toxicity (FBC, U&E, LFT, lactate, blood glucose) and offered a detailed scan to detect fetal anomalies potentially attributable to teratogenesis.

## 9.42 Answers

**A** False.
**B** True.
**C** True.
**D** True.

Note:
• Symptoms/signs of pre-eclampsia, cholestasis or other signs of liver dysfunction may indicate drug toxicity.
• Lactic acidosis is a recognized complication of some HAART regimens – symptoms include GI disturbance, fatigue, fever and SOB. Other side effects include rash, glucose intolerance and hepatotoxicity.

## 9.43 Answers

**A** **True** – Advanced maternal HIV disease, low antenatal CD4 count and high plasma viral load are associated with increased risk of vertical transmission – viral load being the strongest predictor.

**B** **False.**

**C** **True.**

**D** **True** – Obstetric risk factors for vertical transmission include vaginal delivery, duration of membrane rupture, chorioamnionitis, preterm delivery. Breastfeeding is associated with a two-fold increase in vertical transmission rate.

## 9.44 Answers

**A** **True** – CD4 count falls during pregnancy and returns to pre-pregnancy levels post-partum – this is not, however, associated with acceleration of HIV disease or a worsening of prognosis.

**B** **False.**

**C** **False** – There is insufficient evidence for a plasma viral load below which vertical transmission does not occur – transmission has been reported with viral load <1000 copies/ml.

**D** **False** – <2% of vertical transmission occurs in the first/second trimesters. 80% of vertical transmission occurs from 36 weeks onwards, including labour and delivery.

## 9.45 Answers

**A** **True.**

**B** **True.**

**C** **False.**

**D** **False** – A woman with shingles should be immune to chickenpox.

Note:
- Vaccines safe in pregnancy: inactivated virus vaccines – polio (Salk), influenza, rabies, hepatitis A; subunit – hepatitis B, influenza; toxoid – tetanus, diphtheria (vaccination will not cause fetal infection).
- Live attenuated virus vaccines – not safe for use in pregnancy: MMR – measles, mumps, rubella, polio (Sabin), varicella zoster (not in general use), adenovirus, yellow fever.

## 9.46 Answers

**A** **True** – Chorioretinitis.

**B** **True** – Chorioretinitis.

**C** **False** – Not teratogenic.

**D** **True** – Chorioretinitis, optic atrophy.

**9.47** **Answers**

**A** **True** – HPV (juvenile laryngeal papillomatosis) and HIV may be acquired during vaginal delivery.

**B** **True.**

**C** **False** – Early-onset neonatal listeriosis is due to transplacental passage while late-onset disease is horizontally acquired as maternal cultures are usually negative.

**D** **False** – All four species of *Plasmodium* can cause congenital malaria due to transplacental spread – more common with *P. malariae* but malaria is not transmitted as a result of vaginal delivery.

# 10. Urogynaecology and menopause: Questions

10.1 A 57-year-old woman complains of stress incontinence, urinary frequency and urgency:

A A bladder capacity of 200 ml on cystometry is normal.
B Detrusor instability is a possible diagnosis.
C A residual urine volume of 30 ml is normal.
D Peak urine flow rate of 20 ml/s suggests voiding dysfunction.

10.2 In a woman with voiding dysfunction:

A The maximum urinary flow rate is >15 ml/s.
B Urethral pressure is low.
C Detrusor voiding pressure is high.
D Suprapubic catheterization carries a higher risk of urinary tract infection.

10.3 The following urinary symptoms or findings should prompt further investigation/treatment:

A An 80-year-old woman waking up twice at night to pass urine.
B Bladder capacity of 500 ml at cystometry.
C Cough-induced detrusor contraction at cystometry in a woman complaining of stress incontinence.
D Residual urine of 85 ml.

10.4 With respect to the urethra:

A The female urethra is 4–5 cm long.
B The external urethral sphincter is made of smooth muscle.
C The external urethral sphincter is innervated by the pudendal nerve.
D The urethra is lined by transitional epithelium throughout its length.

10.5 The following can precipitate or exacerbate stress incontinence:

A Chronic obstructive airway disease.
B Chronic constipation.
C The alpha-adrenergic agonist phenylpropanolamine.
D Anterior colporrhaphy.

231

10.6 In a 40-year-old woman with genuine stress incontinence and a cystocele:

A Colposuspension has a better short-term success rate than the Marshall–Marchetti–Kantz procedure.
B Colposuspension is adequate treatment for cystocele.
C Colposuspension is associated with an increased risk of enterocele.
D Osteitis pubis is a recognized complication of colposuspension.

10.7 The Burch colposuspension:

A The proximal urethra is elevated to the ipsilateral ileopectineal ligament.
B The parietal peritoneum is opened to access the cave of Retzius.
C Has an 80–90% objective cure rate at 1 year.
D Carries a 1% risk of postoperative de novo detrusor instability.

10.8 Duloxetine:

A Is contraindicated in pregnancy.
B Is not contraindicated during breastfeeding.
C Is associated with nausea and decreased libido.
D Enhances the anticoagulant effects of warfarin.

10.9 Duloxetine:

A Should be stopped immediately if the woman complains of anorgasmia.
B Can be prescribed safely in women treated with selective serotonin re-uptake inhibitors.
C Is an anticholinergic agent.
D Is effective treatment for stress urinary incontinence.

10.10 A 40-year-old woman complains of urinary frequency, urgency and urge incontinence but no other symptoms. The following are effective treatment:

A Oxybutynin.
B Phenylpropanolamine.
C Tolterodine.
D Trospium chloride.

10.11 A 57-year-old woman complains of urinary frequency, urgency and nocturnal enuresis but no other symptoms. The following are effective treatment:

A Imipramine.
B Propantheline bromide.
C Carbachol.
D Phenylpropanolamine.

10.12 The following are recognized causes of vesicovaginal fistula:
A Diverticulosis of the colon.
B Interstitial cystitis.
C Carcinoma of the cervix.
D Carcinoma of the bladder.

10.13 Regarding the mechanism of action of oestrogen:

A The oestrogen receptor is located on the cell membrane.
B There are at least two subtypes of oestrogen receptors – type I and type II.
C The binding of oestrogen to its receptor results in transcription of oestrogen responsive genes.
D Oestrogen has a negative feedback effect on gonadotrophin production.

10.14 With respect to ovarian function around the time of the menopause:

A Ovarian inhibin stimulates FSH release.
B Ovarian sensitivity to gonadotrophins decreases.
C FSH levels are of diagnostic use in a woman with hot flushes.
D Peri-menopausal women taking sequential HRT do not require additional contraception.

10.15 The following are haematological effects of HRT:

A Increased Factors VII and VIII.
B Increased protein C.
C Decreased antithrombin III.
D Decreased protein S.

10.16 The following are recognized causes of premature menopause:
A Down syndrome.
B Turner's syndrome.
C Galactosaemia.
D Chemotherapy.

10.17 With respect to bone density:

A Peak bone density is reached at the age of 40 years in women.
B Loss of bone density occurs at a constant rate after the menopause.
C Smoking is associated with decreased bone density.
D Use of depo-provera is associated with increased bone density.

10.18 The following are risk factors for osteoporosis:

A Low body mass index.
B Alcohol abuse.
C First-degree relative with osteoporosis.
D Chronic liver disease.

10.19 The menopause is associated with:

A Increased risk of urinary tract infections.
B Decreased risk of vaginal infections.
C Increased risk of depressive illness.
D Increased insulin resistance.

10.20 The following oestrogens confer protection against osteoporosis:

A Oestradiol 1 mg daily orally.
B Oestradiol 50 mg implant every 12 months.
C Conjugated equine oestrogen 0.625 mg daily orally.
D Oestradiol patch 25 μg daily.

10.21 For the purpose of oestrogen replacement, the following routes are effective:

A Nasal spray.
B Vaginal rings.
C Intrauterine.
D Transdermal gels.

10.22 Tamoxifen:

A Has antioestrogenic effects on the reproductive tract in pre-menopausal women.
B Is associated with amenorhoea in pre-menopausal women.
C Is associated with increased serum oestradiol levels in pre-menopausal women.
D Is associated with increased serum LDL cholesterol.

10.23 Tamoxifen:

A Is associated with increased hepatic production of sex hormone binding globulin.
B Is associated with decreased hepatic synthesis of thyroxine binding globulin.
C Is associated with ovarian cysts in pre-menopausal women.
D Is associated with a reduction in the risk of benign endometrial pathology.

10.24 In post-menopausal women undergoing major elective surgery:

A HRT should be discontinued 6 weeks preoperatively.
B Raloxifene should be discontinued 3 days preoperatively.
C Tamoxifen should be discontinued because of the increased risk of DVT.
D Endometrial cancer is an absolute contraindication to subsequent HRT.

10.25 With respect to the long-term risks and benefits of HRT:

A There is an increased risk of hypertension.
B There is a significant reduction in the risk of myocardial infarction in women with a previous infarct.
C There is a significant increase in the risk of myocardial infarction in the first year of treatment in women with a previous infarct.
D The risk of gallbladder disease is reduced.

10.26 Tibolone:

A Is a weakly androgenic oestrogen.
B Is administered with progestogens for endometrial protection.
C Relieves vasomotor symptoms.
D Is effective in the prevention of osteoporosis.

10.27 Raloxifene:

A Relieves menopausal symptoms.
B Is associated with an increased risk of venous thromboembolism.
C Stimulates endometrial oestrogen receptors.
D Has been shown to significantly reduce the risk of hip fractures.

10.28 The following drugs are recognized options in the treatment of menopausal women with hot flushes:

A Norethisterone 5 mg daily.
B Raloxifene 60 mg daily.
C Paroxetine.
D Megestrol acetate 40 mg daily.

10.29 With respect to HRT and breast cancer:

A Oestrogen + progestogen HRT is associated with a lower risk of breast cancer compared to oestrogen-only HRT.
B Tibolone is not associated with an increased risk of breast cancer.
C Use of HRT is associated with increased risk of mortality from breast cancer.
D Past use of HRT is associated with an increased risk of developing breast cancer.

10.30 In post-menopausal women with a previous hysterectomy, short-term use of conjugated equine oestrogen is associated with:

A Increased risk of coronary artery disease.
B Increased risk of stroke.
C Increased risk of breast cancer.
D Decreased risk of hip fracture.

10.31 In post-menopausal women with a previous hysterectomy, short-term use of conjugated equine oestrogen is associated with:

A Increased mortality.
B Decreased risk of pulmonary embolism.
C Decreased risk of colorectal cancer.
D A significant reduction in the risk of chronic disease.

10.32 Women who develop breast cancer while taking continuous combined HRT:

A Have smaller tumours.
B Have more advanced disease.
C Are less likely to have metastatic disease.
D Are more likely to have papillary and mucinous tumours.

**10.33** Use of St John's wort is associated with:

A Amenorrhoea.
B Breakthrough bleeding on COCP.
C Failure of COCP.
D Increased plasma concentration of warfarin.

**10.34** The following have been shown to be effective in the relief of vasomotor menopausal symptoms:

A Ginseng.
B Venlafaxine.
C Fluoxetine.
D Oral clonidine.

**10.35** The following have been shown to be effective in the relief of vasomotor menopausal symptoms:

A Transdermal clonidine.
B Vitamin E supplementation.
C Megestrol.
D Raloxifene.

# Answers

### 10.1 Answers

**A** **False** – A bladder capacity of 400–600 ml is normal.

**B** **True** – Detrusor instability can present with stress incontinence, frequency and urgency.

**C** **True** – A residual volume of <50 ml is normal.

**D** **False** – Peak urine flow rate <15 ml/s suggests voiding dysfunction.

### 10.2 Answers

**A** **False** – Normal peak urine flow rate >15 ml/s, lower in voiding dysfunction.

**B** **False** – Urethral pressure is high.

**C** **True.**

**D** **False** – Suprapubic catheterization is associated with a lower risk of UTI compared to urethral catheterization.

### 10.3 Answers

**A** **False** – Frequency of nocturia increases with age. Above 60 years, one episode of nocturia per decade of life is not abnormal.

**B** **False** – See 10.1A.

**C** **True** – Cough-induced detrusor contraction is consistent with detrusor instability.

**D** **True** – See 10.1D.

### 10.4 Answers

**A** **True.**

**B** **False** – External urethral sphincter is made of skeletal muscle of the pelvic floor and the urogenital diaphragm and is supplied by the pudendal nerve.

**C** **True.**

**D** **False** – The urethra is lined by transitional epithelium except in its distal aspect, where it is lined by stratified squamous epithelium.

### 10.5 Answers

**A** **True** – Chronic chest disease, constipation and abdomino-pelvic mass can precipitate or exacerbate stress incontinence.

**B** **True.**

**C** **False** – Alpha-adrenergic agent phenylpropanolamine may be effective treatment for GSI.

**D** **True** – Anterior repair may unmask stress incontinence.

## 10.6 Answers

A **False** – Burch colposuspension – Continence rates of 85–90% at 1 year and 70% at 5 years. Similar success rates to MMK procedure. Success rate lower if previous continence surgery.

B **True.**

C **True.**

D **False.**

Note: Complications of colposuspension:
- De novo detrusor instability – 17% (8–27%).
- Voiding dysfunction – 10% (2–27%).
- Enterocoele and/or rectocele formation – 14% (3–27%) after 5 years.
- The most significant complication of the Marshall–Marchetti Krantz (MMK) procedure is the development of osteitis pubis (2.5% risk).

## 10.7 Answers

A **False** – The Burch colposuspension elevates the paravaginal tissue to the ipsilateral ileopectineal ligament.

B **False** – The cave of Retzius is extraperitoneal.

C **True** – Continence rates of 85–90% at 1 year and 70% at 5 years.

D **False** – Risk of de novo detrusor instability is 17% (8–27%).

## 10.8 Answers

A **True.**

B **False.**

C **True.**

D **True.**

## 10.9 Answers

A **False** – Withdrawal reaction is characterized by headache, nausea, paraesthesia, dizziness and anxiety – drug should not be stopped abruptly and dose should be reduced over a 2-week period.

B **False.**

C **True** – Combined serotonin and noradrenaline re-uptake inhibitor. Increased synaptic concentrations of noradrenaline and 5-HT within the pudendal nerve results in increased stimulation of the urethral sphincter.

D **True.**

Note:
- Duloxitine increases sphincter activity in the storage phase of the micturiction cycle.
- Side effects: GI disturbance particularly nausea and dry mouth, headache, decreased libido, anorgasmia.
- Contraindications: pregnancy, lactation, hepatic impairment, monoamine oxidase therapy, lowers seizure threshold therefore avoid in epilepsy.
- Interactions: can enhance the anticoagulant effects of warfarin. Metabolized by the same enzymes as ciprofloxacin and fluvoxamine – avoid co-prescription. Avoid co-prescription with SSRIs and tricyclic antidepressants.

### 10.10 Answers

**A** True.
**B** False – Phenylpropanolamine is an alpha-adrenergic agonist which may be useful in GSI.
**C** True.
**D** True.

Note:

- Anticholinergic agents: oxybutynin, tolterodine, propiverine, trospium chloride – improvement in 57–71% of women; significant placebo effect and side effects.

### 10.11 Answers

**A** True – Tricyclic antidepressants – anticholinergic effects and also sedative; useful in nocturia and nocturnal enuresis. Main side effects are drowsiness and postural hypotension.
**B** True – Popantheleine bromide is rarely used as it has a low response rate and a high incidence of side effects. Useful for adult enuresis.
**C** False – Carbachol is a parasympathomimetic which is rarely used for urinary retention.
**D** False.

### 10.12 Answers

**A** False.
**B** False.
**C** True.
**D** True.

Note: Causes of vesicovaginal fistula:

- Commonest cause worldwide is obstructed labour.
- Surgical trauma – vaginal repair, hysterectomy, C/S.
- Pelvic malignancy – direct invasion or post-radiotherapy.

### 10.13 Answers

**A** False – The oestrogen receptor is a nuclear transcription factor which dimerizes and undergoes conformational change on oestrogen binding.
**B** False – Two oestrogen receptor (ER) subtypes have been described – ER-$\alpha$ and ER-$\beta$. The differential distribution of these receptor subtypes in tissues and their differential binding to oestrogen receptor modulators underlies the therapeutic use of drugs to target specific oestrogen-sensitive tissues.
**C** True – The oestrogen bound receptor dimer interacts with oestrogen response elements within the promoter region of oestrogen-responsive genes, initiating transcription.
**D** True – Oestrogen has a negative feedback effect on pituitary gonadotrophin production.

## 10.14 Answers

**A False** – Ovarian inhibin inhibits pituitary FSH secretion.

**B True** – The ovaries become less responsive to gonadotrophins several years before cessation of menstruation, resulting in a progressive rise in gonadotrophin levels.

**C False** – FSH levels fluctuate markedly from pre- to post-menopausal levels on a daily basis during the menopausal transition and measurement is therefore of very limited diagnostic value.

**D False** – Sequential HRT is not contraceptive and appropriate contraception should be recommended in peri-menopausal women.

## 10.15 Answers

**A** True.
**B** True.
**C** True.
**D** True.

Note:

- Associated with increased protein C, Factors VII and VIII, and decreased fibrinogen, antithrombin III and protein S.
- C-reactive protein also increases with oestrogen-containing HRT and CRP is a marker for cardiovascular risk including VTE.
- Also associated with increased resistance to protein C.

## 10.16 Answers

**A** True.
**B** True.
**C** True.
**D** True.

Note: Causes of premature ovarian failure:

- Autoimmune condition associated with other autoimmune disorders such as thyroid disease, parathyroid and adrenal insufficiency.
- Iatrogenic – surgery/chemotherapy/irradiation.
- Chromosomal abnormalities – Turner's syndrome including mosaics, gonadal dysgenesis. Down syndrome is associated with premature ovarian failure.
- Metabolic disorders including galactosaemia (toxic effect of galactose metabolites on germ cell migration), 17-hydroxylase deficiency.
- Infections – pelvic TB, mumps.
- Environmental causes – smoking.
- Idiopathic.

## 10.17 Answers

**A** **False** – Peak bone density is reached during the 20s.

**B** **False** – Peak bone density declines from the mid-40s onwards, with an accelerated period of decline for 6–10 years after the menopause, followed by a period of slower bone loss.

**C** **True** – See 10.18.

**D** **False** – Depo-provera is associated with anovulation and a theoretical risk of hypo-oestrogenaemia and osteopaenia.

## 10.18 Answers

**A** **True.**

**B** **True.**

**C** **True.**

**D** **True.**

Note:

• Risk of osteoporosis is dependent on peak bone density, rate of loss and life-span.
• Other risk factors include family history, smoking and alcohol use, immobility, corticosteroids, hyperthyroidism, hypogonadism, chronic liver disease, malabsorption and low vitamin D intake. Osteoporosis is less common in Afro-Caribbean compared to Caucasians.

## 10.19 Answers

**A** **True.**

**B** **False** – There is an increased risk of vaginal infections.

**C** **False** – The association between psychological symptoms such as depressed mood, anxiety, irritability, lack of energy, loss of memory and lack of concentration and the menopause, or specifically oestrogen deficiency, is controversial.

**D** **True** – The menopause is associated with an increase in body mass index and increased insulin resistance.

Note:

• Urogenital symptoms of the menopause – vaginal dryness and dyspareunia; urinary frequency, dysuria, nocturia, urgency and incontinence.

## 10.20 Answers

**A** **True** – Minimum bone-sparing dose of oral oestradiol: 1–2 mg daily.

**B** **False** – Oestradiol implant: 50 mg every 6 months.

**C** **True** – Conjugated equine oestrogen: 0.3–0.625 mg daily.

**D** **True** – Oestradiol patch: 25–50 μg daily.

Note:

• Oestardiol gel: 1–5 g (depends on preparation).

## 10.21 Answers

A True.
B True.
C False.
D True.

Note:
* Oestrogen replacement may be administered by the oral route, implants, gels, patches, vaginal rings/pesseries/tablets, nasal sprays.

## 10.22 Answers

A **True** – Antioestrogenic effects in reproductive tract of pre-menopausal women; oestrogenic effects in post-menopausal women.
B **True** – Hypothalamic–pituitary–ovarian axis: pre-menopausal women – tamoxifen acts as an antioestrogen, resulting in increased ovarian steroid synthesis and irregular cycles. Amenorrhoea in ~25% of women.
C **True**.
D **False** – Associated with a reduction in serum cholesterol and LDL cholesterol in post-menopausal women.

Note:
* Serum gonadotrophin levels are unchanged.

## 10.23 Answers

A **True** – Associated with increased hepatic synthesis of sex hormone, thyroxine and cortisol-binding globulins.
B **False** – Free thyroxine and TSH levels are unchanged.
C **True** – ~10% risk of ovarian cysts.
D **False**.

Note:
* A case–control study has shown that the risk of endometrial cancer is increased with longer duration of tamoxifen use, with relative risks of 2.0 (1.2–3.2) for 2–5 years and 6.9 (2.4–19.4) for at least 5 years compared with non-users.
* Endometrial cancers of stage III and IV occurred more frequently in long-term tamoxifen users (≥2 years) than in non-users (17.4% vs 5.4%).
* Long-term users were more likely than non-users to have had malignant mixed mesodermal tumours or sarcomas of the endometrium (15.4% vs 2.9%).

## 10.24 Answers

A **False** – HRT should not be routinely stopped but should be considered during risk assessment for thromboprophylaxis.
B **True** – Raloxifene should be discontinued 3 days before major elective surgery – three-fold increase in VTE risk.
C **False** – Tamoxifen should not be discontinued before major surgery.
D **False** – The effect of HRT in women with a history of endometrial cancer remains uncertain.

## 10.25 Answers

**A** **False** – No evidence that HRT is associated with increased risk of hypertension.

**B** **False** – In women with established coronary artery disease, the available evidence indicates that overall, HRT does not confer an advantage and is associated with an increased risk of coronary artery events in the first year.

**C** **True** – In women without cardiovascular disease, the WHI trial showed that continuous combined HRT is associated with an increased risk of coronary heart disease: relative risk 1.29 (1.02–1.63), stroke: relative risk 1.41 (1.07–1.85), and pulmonary embolism: relative risk 2.13 (1.39–3.25).

**D** **False** – The risk of gallbladder disease is increased.

## 10.26 Answers

**A** **True** – Has oestrogenic, progestogenic and weak androgenic activity.

**B** **False** – As tibolone has progestogenic activity, progestogens are not required for endometrial protection.

**C** **True.**

**D** **True.**

## 10.27 Answers

**A** **False** – Does not relieve vasomotor menopausal symptoms.

**B** **True** – Associated with an increased risk of venous thromboembolism (relative risk 3.1).

**C** **False** – Antioestrogenic effects on reproductive tract.

**D** **False** – Osteo-protective and associated with increased bone mineral density and a significant reduction in vertebral fractures in osteoporotic women. There is a non-significant reduction in non-vertebral fractures.

## 10.28 Answers

**A** **True.**

**B** **False** – SERMS (selective oestrogen receptor modulators) such as raloxifene are *not* effective.

**C** **True.**

**D** **True.**

Note: Treatments for hot flushes:

- Oestrogens.
- Progestogens – norethisterone 5 mg daily, megestrol acetate 40 mg daily.
- SSRIs (selective serotonin reuptake inhibitors) such as venlaflaxine and paroxetine.
- Propranolol – efficacy is doubtful.
- Clonidine – efficacy limited.

## 10.29 Answers

    **A** **False** – Incidence of breast cancer is significantly increased for current users of preparations containing oestrogen only (1.30 [1.21–1.40], P< 0.0001), oestrogen-progestogen (2.00 [1.88–2.12], P< 0.0001), and tibolone (1.45 [1.25–1.68], P< 0.0001).

    **B** **False.**

    **C** **True** – Current users of HRT are more likely to die from breast cancer (adjusted relative risk 1.22 [1.00–1.48], p = 0.05).

    **D** **False** – Past users of HRT are not at an increased risk of developing breast cancer (1.01 [0.94–1.09] or dying from it (1.05 [0.82–1.34]).

## 10.30 Answers

    **A** **False** – Conjugated equine oestrogen did not affect CHD incidence in postmenopausal women with prior hysterectomy over an average of 6.8 years.

    **B** **True.**

    **C** **False** – A possible reduction in breast cancer risk requires further investigation.

    **D** **True.**

Note:

- The burden of incident disease events was equivalent in the conjugated equine estrogen and placebo groups, indicating no overall benefit.

## 10.31 Answers

    **A** **False.**

    **B** **False.**

    **C** **False.**

    **D** **False.**

Note:

- Estimated hazard ratios (95% confidence intervals) for conjugated equine oestrogen vs placebo for the major clinical outcomes were (WHI Trial): coronary heart disease, 0.91 (0.75–1.12) with 376 cases; breast cancer, 0.77 (0.59–1.01) with 218 cases; stroke, 1.39 (1.10–1.77) with 276 cases; PE, 1.34 (0.87–2.06) with 85 cases; colorectal cancer, 1.08 (0.75–1.55) with 119 cases; hip fracture, 0.61 (0.41–0.91) with 102 cases.
- Corresponding results for composite outcomes were: total cardiovascular disease, 1.12 (1.01–1.24); total cancer, 0.93 (0.81–1.07); total fractures, 0.70 (0.63–0.79); total mortality, 1.04 (0.88–1.22); global index, 1.01 (0.91–1.12).

## 10.32 Answers

**A** False.
**B** True.
**C** False.
**D** False.

Note: Breast cancer risk with HRT (WHI trial):

* Oestrogen plus progestogen increased total (245 vs 185 cases; hazard ratio [HR], 1.24; weighted $P < 0.001$) and invasive (199 vs 150 cases; HR, 1.24; weighted $P = 0.003$) breast cancers compared with placebo.
* The invasive breast cancers diagnosed in the oestrogen plus progestogen group were similar in histology and grade but were larger (mean [SD], 1.7 cm [1.1] vs 1.5 cm [0.9], respectively; $P = 0.04$) and were at a more advanced stage (regional/metastatic 25.4% vs 16.0%, respectively; $P = 0.04$) compared with those diagnosed in the placebo group.
* After 1 year, the percentage of women with abnormal mammograms was substantially greater in the oestrogen plus progestogen group (716 [9.4%] of 7656) compared with placebo group (398 [5.4%] of 7310; $P < 0.001$), a pattern which continued for the study duration.

## 10.33 Answers

**A** False.
**B** True – Can cause COCP failure and breakthrough bleeding.
**C** True.
**D** False.

Note:

* St John's wort is effective in the treatment of mild–moderate depressive illness.
* Efficacy in treatment of menopausal symptoms is unproven.
* Has potentially serious interactions with cyclosporine, tacrolimus, digoxin, midazolam, warfarin, indinavir and theophylline (reduces plasma concentrations).

## 10.34 Answers

**A** False – Ginseng is ineffective in the treatment of menopausal symptoms, although it is associated with improved feeling of well-being and relief of depression.
**B** True – SNRI venlafaxine appears to be most effective agent.
**C** True – Both SSRIs (fluoxetine, paroxetine) and SNRIs have been shown to be effective in the treatment of hot flushes.
**D** False – Evidence is that oral clonidine is ineffective, while transdermal clonidine is effective in relieving vasomotor symptoms.

## 10.35 Answers

**A** **True** – See 10.34D.

**B** **False** – Dietary supplements such as vitamins C and E and selenium have not been shown to be effective.

**C** **True** – RCT shows modest benefit for megestrol in the relief of vasomotor symptoms.

**D** **False** – ERMs do not relieve menopausal symptoms.

Note:
- The evidence is that evening primrose oil is ineffective in the treatment of hot flushes.
- Exercise – aerobic, sustained, regular exercise associated with an improvement in menopausal symptoms. Infrequent, high-impact exercise may exacerbate symptoms.
- Acupuncture has been shown to be effective in the relief of hot flushes in a small randomized trial.

# 11. Endocrinology and reproduction: Questions

**11.1** With respect to endocrine changes around the time of puberty:

A LH and FSH levels are elevated in the pre-pubertal female.
B GnRH levels are elevated in the pre-pubertal female.
C The increase in pulse frequency and pulse amplitude of LH secretion occurs initially during sleep at puberty.
D A positive feedback response of gonadotrophins to rising oestrogen levels induces ovulation.

**11.2** During the development of secondary sexual characteristics:

A Breast development begins before the development of axillary hair.
B Breast development is divided into five stages.
C Axillary hair development occurs in five stages.
D Pubic hair development occurs in three stages.

**11.3** The following are recognized causes of delayed menarche/primary amenorrhoea:

A Androgen insensitivity syndrome.
B Ovarian granulosa cell tumour.
C Craniopharingioma.
D Low vaginal atresia.

**11.4** The following are likely diagnoses in a 16-year-old woman with primary amenorrhoea but normal breast, pubic and axillary hair development:

A Androgen insensitivity syndrome.
B Uterine agenesis.
C Kallman's syndrome.
D Congenital adrenal hyperplasia.

11.5 The following are likely diagnoses in a 16-year-old woman with primary amenorrhoea and raised LH and FSH levels:

A Turner's syndrome.
B Kallman's syndrome.
C Rokitanski's syndrome.
D Ovarian agenesis.

11.6 The following are likely diagnoses in a 16-year-old with primary amenorrhoea and raised LH and FSH levels:

A Craniopharingioma.
B Ovarian failure secondary to chemotherapy.
C Asherman's syndrome.
D Galactosaemia.

11.7 The following groups of women with primary amenorrhoea can have children of their own (including surrogacy):

A Kallman's syndrome.
B Rokitanski's syndrome.
C Ovarian agenesis.
D Androgen insensitivity syndrome.

11.8 The following diagnoses are likely in a 30-year-old woman with secondary amenorrhoea and low gonadotrophin levels:

A Premature ovarian failure.
B Resistant ovary syndrome.
C Sheehan's syndrome.
D Prolactin-secreting pituitary adenoma.

11.9 The following are characteristic of Turner's syndrome:

A Secondary amenorrhoea.
B Hypergonadotrophic hypogonadism.
C Short stature.
D Streak ovaries.

11.10 Anorexia nervosa:

A Is associated with hypothermia and tachycardia.
B Typically affects women before the age of 25 years.
C Is associated with weight loss >25% of original body weight.
D May present with primary amenorrhoea.

11.11 Androgen insensitivity syndrome:

A Is typically due to 5-alpha-reductase deficiency.
B Typically presents at puberty with primary amenorrhoea.
C Is associated with a 46,XX karyotype.
D The uterus and fallopian tubes are usually present.


11.12 With respect to the androgen insensitivity syndrome:

A Normal breast development occurs.
B There is normal development of axillary and pubic hair.
C Fertility is possible with ovulation induction.
D Secondary amenorrhoea may be the presenting complaint.


11.13 5-alpha reductase deficiency:

A Is an autosomal recessive disorder.
B Is associated with impaired development of Wolffian duct structures.
C Is associated with poor masculinization of the external genitalia.
D Is associated with an increased risk of malignancy in the gonads.


11.14 The following are characteristic features of congenital adrenal hyperplasia:

A Clitoral enlargement.
B Precocious puberty.
C Absent uterus and fallopian tubes in a 46,XX neonate.
D Vomiting and failure to thrive in the neonatal period.


11.15 The polycystic ovary syndrome:

A Is associated with LH hypersecretion.
B Is associated with low TSH levels.
C Typically presents with primary amenorrhoea.
D Is associated with increased production of DHEA-sulphate, an adrenal androgen.

11.16 The polycystic ovary syndrome:

A Is associated with markedly elevated serum prolactin.
B Occurs in 20% of women of reproductive age.
C Accounts for 20% of cases of anovulatory infertility.
D With hypersecretion of LH is associated with a reduced chance of continuing a pregnancy.

11.17 The following are inconsistent with a diagnosis of the polycystic ovary syndrome:

A Normal ovarian morphology on ultrasound scan.
B LH:FSH ratio <2:1.
C Normal body mass index.
D Rapidly progressive virilization.

11.18 In the management of anovulatory infertility in a woman with the polycystic ovary syndrome:

A The recommended duration of use of gonadotrophin therapy is 6–12 months.
B Laparoscopic ovarian diathermy is associated with the same risk of adhesion formation as wedge resection.
C Laparoscopic ovarian diathermy is associated with an increased risk of multiple pregnancy.
D Downregulation of LH hypersecretion has been shown to significantly improve pregnancy outcome.

11.19 With respect to the management of anovulatory infertility in a woman with polycystic ovary syndrome:

A Laparoscopic ovarian drilling is more effective than gonadotrophin therapy in women who are clomiphene resistant.
B Laparoscopic ovarian drilling is associated with the ovarian hyperstimulation syndrome.
C Ultrasound follicular tracking is unnecessary in women treated with laparoscopic ovarian drilling.
D Lararoscopic ovarian drilling is associated with a normalization of LH levels.

**11.20** In women with anovulatory infertility secondary to the polycystic ovary syndrome:

A Recombinant FSH is effective ovulation induction therapy.
B Human menopausal gonadotrophin is effective ovulation induction therapy.
C The routine use of GnRH analogues in conjunction with gonadotrophins is associated with increased pregnancy rates.
D There is an increased risk of first trimester miscarriage.

**11.21** The following are long-term consequences of the polycystic ovary syndrome

A Increased mortality from cardiovascular disease.
B Increased risk of ovarian cancer.
C Increased risk of endometrial cancer.
D Increased risk of insulin-dependent diabetes mellitus.

**11.22** The following are recognized clinical manifestations of the polycystic ovary syndrome:

A Acanthosis nigricans.
B Obesity.
C Acne.
D Recurrent miscarriage.

**11.23** The polycystic ovary syndrome is associated with:

A Increased levels of sex hormone binding globulin.
B Decreased levels of biologically active oestradiol.
C Increased ovarian production of DHEA-sulphate.
D Increased ovarian production of androstendione.

**11.24** In women with PCOS, treatment with metformin is associated with:

A Significant weight loss
B Ovarian hyperstimulation syndrome
C Increased risk of multiple pregnancy
D Increased fasting insulin concentration

**11.25** In women with PCOS, treatment with metformin is associated with:

A Decreased systolic and diastolic blood pressure.
B Decreased total cholesterol concentration.
C Increased nausea and vomiting.
D No increase in ovulation rate in women who are clomiphene resistant.

11.26 Laparoscopic ovarian drilling in the management of polycystic ovary syndrome:

A Is associated with normalization of serum androgen levels.
B Is associated with a reduction in sex hormone binding globulin levels.
C Is not associated with ovarian hyperstimulation.
D Is associated with a reduction in the risk of NIDDM in later life.

11.27 In a 30-year-old nulliparous woman with obesity and a diagnosis of polycystic ovary syndrome:

A A glucose tolerance test should be recommended on a yearly basis.
B Serum lipid profile should be performed.
C Metformin can be expected to reduce the risk of developing NIDDM in future.
D Metformin can be expected to result in increased insulin resistance in the short term.

11.28 With respect to androgen production in the female:

A Testosterone is the main adrenal androgen.
B Androstendione is the main ovarian androgen.
C Androstendione and dehydroepiandrosterone do not have direct androgenic activity.
D Dehydroepiandrosterone sulphate is almost exclusively of adrenal origin.

11.29 With respect to androgen activity in the female:

A Testosterone bound to SHBG is biologically inactive.
B Testosterone bound to albumin is biologically inactive.
C Increased 5-alpha-reductase activity may lead to signs of hyperandrogenism.
D Androstendione is converted to testosterone in peripheral tissue.

11.30 The following ovarian tumours are associated with hyperandrogenism:

A Sertoli–Leydig cell tumours.
B Hilus cell tumours.
C Luteomas.
D Yolk sac tumours.

**11.31** A 30-year-old woman presents with rapidly progressive hirsutism and virilization:

A Ovarian hilus cell tumour is a possible diagnosis.
B A tumour of the adrenal medulla is a possible cause.
C Excision of an androgen-producing ovarian tumour results in a rapid regression of hirsutism.
D Polycystic ovary syndrome is a possible diagnosis.

**11.32** The following drugs are associated with hirsutism:
A Danazol.
B Phenytoin.
C Cyclosporine A.
D Norethisterone.

**11.33** With respect to drug treatment for hirsutism:

A The combined oral contraceptive pill reduces SHBG production.
B The combined oral contraceptive pill reduces LH production.
C Medroxyprogesterone acetate reduces LH production.
D Progestogens inhibit 5-alpha-reductase activity.

**11.34** With respect to drug treatment for hirsutism:

A Spironolactone is associated with hypertension and hyperkalaemia.
B Flutamide is a 5-alpha-reductase inhibitor.
C Finasteride is a testosterone antagonist.
D Cyproterone acetate is a progestogen.

**11.35** In a 24-year-old sexually active woman who is not using any contraception, the following are suitable treatments for acne:

A Oral tetracycline.
B Cyproterone acetate.
C Isotrentinion.
D Topical benzoly peroxide.

**11.36** The following are recognized side effects of clomiphene citrate:

A Visual disturbance.
B Hair loss.
C Hot flushes.
D Postural hypotension.

**11.37** The following side effects are associated with the drugs listed:

A Jaundice – cyproterone acetate.
B Fatigue – cyproterone acetate.
C Breast tenderness and enlargement – finasteride.
D Visual disturbance – tamoxifen.

**11.38** The following are recognized causes of secondary amenorrhoea:

A Excessive weight loss.
B Excessive exercise.
C Androgen insensitivity syndrome.
D Prolactin-secreting adenoma.

**11.39** Prolactin:

A Is a polypeptide hormone.
B Is produced by posterior pituitary lactotrophs.
C Is produced by the endometrium.
D Is produced by decidua.

**11.40** The following conditions are associated with mildly elevated serum prolactin:

A Stress.
B Breast stimulation.
C Prolactin secreting macroadenoma.
D Polycystic ovary syndrome.

**11.41** The following drugs are associated with hyperprolactinaemia:

A Opiates.
B Phenothiazines.
C L-Dopa.
D Metoclopramide.

**11.42** The following are associated with hyperprolactinaemia:

A Shingles affecting the intercostal nerves.
B Thoracic surgery.
C Chronic renal disease.
D Anorexia nervosa.

**11.43** A 30-year-old woman with primary infertility and hyperprolacti-naemia is found to have a pituitary microadenoma:

A Carbegolline is an alternative to bromocriptine for ovulation induction.

B Bromocriptine therapy is associated with a reduction in tumour size.

C Prolactin levels should be monitored in pregnancy.

D There is a 50% risk of symptomatic enlargement of the adenoma in pregnancy.

**11.44** A 30-year-old woman with primary infertility and hyperprolacti-naemia is found to have a pituitary macroadenoma:

A The pituitary tumour is <10 mm in diameter.

B There is a 15–30% risk of symptomatic enlargement of the adenoma in pregnancy.

C Trans-sphenoidal surgery is the recommended first-line treatment.

D ACTH and TSH levels may be low.

**11.45** In pregnancy associated with a pituitary macroadenoma:

A Homonymous hemianopia is the typical visual symptom.

B Headache is the earliest symptom of tumour enlargement.

C Bromocriptine should be discontinued.

D Serum prolactin levels are a good indicator of tumour size.

**11.46** The following are typical side effects of bromocriptine therapy:

A Nausea and vomiting.

B Postural hypotension.

C Constipation.

D Tinnitus.

**11.47** Ovarian hyperstimulation syndrome:

A Is associated with hypokalaemic acidosis.

B Is commonly associated with the use of oral ovulation-inducing drugs.

C Is commoner in older than younger women.

D Should be managed with intravenous frusemide if urine output is <20 ml/h.

11.48 Ovarian hyperstimulation syndrome:

A Is less likely to increase in severity if pregnancy ensures.
B In the mild form occurs in 50% of IVF cycles.
C May result in adult respiratory distress syndrome.
D Treatment may include the use of i.v. dextran.

11.49 Kallman's syndrome:

A Is due to failure of development of the gonadotrophin cells of the pituitary gland.
B Is a recognized cause of secondary amenorrhoea.
C Is typically associated with nerve deafness.
D Is an X-linked recessive disorder.

11.50 Secondary amenorrhoea is a recognized feature of:

A Addison's disease.
B Down syndrome.
C Bulimia nervosa.
D Androgen insensitivity syndrome.

11.51 Premature ovarian failure:

A Should be differentiated from the resistant ovary syndrome by ovarian biopsy.
B Serum FSH levels >40 IU/L indicate permanent ovarian failure.
C There is an association with an increased risk of ovarian cancer.
D Is associated with an increased risk of myocardial infarction.

11.52 Premature ovarian failure:

A Is usually associated with an identifiable autoimmune factor.
B Is associated with chromosomal anomalies in <10% of women affected below the age of 30 years.
C Is clinically indistinguishable from the resistant ovary syndrome.
D Has an autoimmune aetiology in over 30% of cases.

# Answers

## 11.1 Answers

**A False** – Pre-pubertal – low circulating LH and FSH: CNS–hypothalamic axis is very sensitive to low levels or circulating oestrogens.
**B False** – Increased GnRH production by the hypothalamus occurs once a critical weight or body composition is attained, causing increased LH and to a lesser extent FSH.
**C True** – Episodic pulses of LH occur initially during sleep and subsequently while awake. Lead to increased gonadal steroid synthesis.
**D True** – Activation of the positive gonadotrophin response to increasing levels of oestradiol results in the mid-cycle gonadotrophin surge and ovulation.

## 11.2 Answers

**A True** – The first sign of puberty is the appearance of breast buds which occurs at ~9 years of age followed within a few months by the appearance of pubic hair. Axillary hair development begins at ~13 years.
**B True.**
**C False.**
**D False.**

Note:
- Secondary sexual characteristics include the development of breasts, pubic and axillary hair.
- Breast and pubic hair development is divided into five stages (Tanner stages 1–5) while axillary hair development has three stages.

## 11.3 Answers

**A True.**
**B False.**
**C True.**
**D True.**

Note: Causes of primary amenorrhoea:
- Abnormal karyotype.
- Abnormal CNS–hypothalamic response.
- Abnormal pituitary function including tumours such as craniopharingioma.
- Gonadal/adrenal abnormalities.
- Abnormal end-organs/end-organ response such as: androgen insensitivity syndrome, 5-alpha-reductase deficiency, vaginal atresia.

## 11.4 Answers

**A** **False** – Androgen insensitivity syndrome – absent/scanty pubic and axillary hair, short blind-ending vagina, absent uterus and cervix.

**B** **True.**

**C** **False** – Kallman's syndrome is characterized by hypogonadism and infantile sexual development.

**D** **True** – Late-onset CAH is also characterized by evidence of hyperandrogenaemia.

## 11.5 Answers

**A** **True.**

**B** **False** – See 11.4C. Gonadotrophins are low in Kallman's syndrome.

**C** **False.**

**D** **True.**

Note: Causes of hypergonadotrophic hypogonadism: post-menopausal, castration, ovarian failure or dysgenesis/agenesis.

## 11.6 Answers

**A** **False** – Gonadotrophin levels are low in craniopharingioma.

**B** **True.**

**C** **False** – Asherman's syndrome is associated with normal gonadotrophins.

**D** **True.**

Note:
- Raised LH and FSH would be secondary to ovarian agenesis/dysgenesis or ovarian failure.

## 11.7 Answers

**A** **True** – Kallman's syndrome: ovaries respond to gonadotrophins and induction of ovulation is possible. Clomiphene is ineffective.

**B** **True** – Rokitanski's syndrome: absent vagina and non-functioning uterus. Ovulation possible with IVF.

**C** **False** – Fertility is not possible.

**D** **False** – 46,XY; fertility is not possible.

## 11.8 Answers

**A** **False** – Gonadotrophin levels would be elevated in premature ovarian failure.

**B** **False** – Gonadotrophin levels would be elevated in resistant ovary syndrome.

**C** **True** – Sheehan's syndrome (post-partum pituitary necrosis) would cause low gonadotrophins.

**D** **True** – Pituitary adenoma would cause low gonadotrophins.

Note:

- Laser or diathermy (four-point diathermy set at 40 W for 4 seconds at each point applied to each ovary) is as effective as routine gonadotrophin therapy for ovulation induction in women with clomiphene-resistant PCOS.

## 11.9 Answers

**A** **False** – Primary amenorrhoea (menstruation may occur in some and pregnancy has been reported).

**B** **True.**

**C** **True.**

**D** **True.**

Note:

- 45X0: There is short stature with no adolescent growth spurt, webbed neck, wide carrying angle, hypoplasia of the nails and short fourth metacarpals, broad chest with widely spaced nipples and a low hair line; associated with peripheral lymphoedema in 40% of cases.
- Streak ovaries with primary amenorrhoea and hypergonadotrophic hypogonadism.
- Increased risk of systemic hypertension and Hashimoto's thyroiditis.
- Normal intellectual development.

## 11.10 Answers

**A** **False** – Associated with lanugo hair, bradycardia, hypotension, constipation, hypothermia, vomiting (may be self-induced) and periods of over-activity.

**B** **True** – Typical onset before the age of 25 years.

**C** **True** – Weight loss >25% original body weight. Distorted body image with implacable attitude towards eating.

**D** **True** – May occur in adolescents and can present with primary amenorrhoea.

Note:

- One of the most important causes of secondary amenorrhoea in adolescents.
- Amenorrhoea frequently pre-dates weight loss.
- Exclude medical illness that could cause weight loss. Exclude other psychiatric disorders.
- Psychiatric referral required.

### 11.11 Answers

**A** **False** – Due to mutations in the gene coding for the androgen receptor.
**B** **True** – Most patients present after puberty.
**C** **False** – 46,XY karyotype.
**D** **False** – Short blind-ending vagina, absent uterus and cervix.

### 11.12 Answers

**A** **True.**
**B** **False** – Absent/scanty pubic and axillary hair.
**C** **False.**
**D** **False.**

Note:

- Testes found within the abdomen, inguinal canal, labia. Increased risk of cancer in testes – gonadectomy recommended after puberty + oestrogen replacement therapy.

### 11.13 Answers

**A** **True.**
**B** **False** – Development of Wolffian duct structures is independent of 5-alpha-reductase.
**C** **True** – Poor masculinization of external genitalia in male fetus.
**D** **False** – Not associated with increased risk of gonadal malignancy.

Note:

- Uterus, tubes and vagina are absent as production of Müllerian inhibitory factor is normal.

### 11.14 Answers

**A** **True** – Clitoral enlargement; fusion of genital folds; thickening and rugosity of the labia majora which resemble the scrotum.
**B** **True** – Syndrome may be unrecognized in the male and later presents with precocious puberty.
**C** **False** – Uterus, fallopian tubes and vagina are always present in females although the introitus may be difficult to identify.
**D** **True** – Salt losing syndrome may present with vomiting and failure to thrive secondary to aldosterone deficiency.

### 11.15 Answers

**A** **True** – LH hypersecretion is found in 40% of women with PCOS and is associated with a reduced chance of conception and increased risk of miscarriage.
**B** **False** – TSH unaffected.
**C** **False** – Typically presents with secondary amenorrhoea.
**D** **True** – About 50% of women with PCOS have elevated levels of DHEA-S.

## 11.16 Answers

**A** **False** – Hyperprolactinaemia – mild and present in ~20% of women with PCOS.

**B** **False** – Affects 5–10% of women in their reproductive years, although PCO found in 16–33% of asymptomatic women.

**C** **False** – Majority of women with anovulatory infertility have PCOS.

**D** **True** – See 11.15A.

## 11.17 Answers

**A** **True** – Women with clinical or biochemical evidence of PCOS but with normal ovarian morphology on ultrasound scan should be considered as having hyperandrogenic chronic anovulation.

**B** **False** – Women with PCOS may have normal LH:FSH ratio.

**C** **False**– Women with PCOS may have a normal BMI.

**D** **True** – Rapidly progressive virilization would indicate an androgen-secreting tumour.

Note:

- PCOS is a biochemically and clinically heterogeneous condition.

## 11.18 Answers

**A** **False** – Recommended duration of use of gonadotrophins should not exceed 6 months.

**B** **False** – Ovarian drilling has now replaced wedge resection, which was associated with extensive peri-ovarian and tubal adhesions.

**C** **False** – LOD is not associated with an increased risk of multiple pregnancy.

**D** **False** – Downregulation of LH hypersecretion does not alter pregnancy outcome.

## 11.19 Answers

**A** **False** – Laparoscopic ovarian drilling is as effective as routine gonadotrophin therapy for ovulation induction in women with clomiphene-resistant PCOS.

**B** **False** – Laparoscopic ovarian drilling is not associated with OHSS and therefore follicular tracking is not required.

**C** **True.**

**D** **True** – Leads to ovulation in 80% of patients with a normalization of LH concentrations, good pregnancy rates (40–69%) and a low miscarriage rate (14% compared to 30–40% for women treated by hormonal ovulation induction).

### 11.20 Answers

**A** **True** – Both recombinant FSH and human menopausal gonadotrophin (hMG) are effective ovulation induction agents in women with clomiphene-resistant PCOS (about 20–30% of women with PCOS).

**B** **True.**

**C** **False** – There is no advantage in routinely using GnRH analogues in conjunction with gonadotrophins in these women: no increase in pregnancy rate and their use may be associated with an increased risk of ovarian hyperstimulation.

**D** **True** – Risk of first trimester miscarriage is increased and this is not reduced by suppression of LH hypersecretion.

### 11.21 Answers

**A** **False.**

**B** **True.**

**C** **True.**

**D** **False.**

Note: Long-term sequelae of PCOS:

- Increased incidence of gestational diabetes.
- Increased incidence of pregnancy-induced hypertension.
- Increased risk of endometrial cancer (5-fold).
- Increased risk of ovarian cancer (2.5-fold).
- Cardiovascular disease – mortality is not significantly increased although women with PCOS have abnormal lipid profiles.
- Increased risk of adult-onset diabetes mellitus (40% risk of NIDDM by the age of 40 years).

### 11.22 Answers

**A** **True.**

**B** **True.**

**C** **True.**

**D** **True.**

Note: Clinical presentation of PCOS:

- Menstrual abnormalities – amenorrhoea/oligomenorrhoea/irregular uterine bleeding secondary to the effects of unopposed oestrogens on the endometrium (30% of patients have a regular menstrual cycle).
- Infertility.
- Obesity.
- Hyperandrogenism – hirsutism, acne, male pattern baldness, acanthosis nigricans.
- Increased risk of recurrent first trimester miscarriage.

## 11.23 Answers

   **A** **False** – Decreased sex hormone binding globulin production by the liver with a resultant increase in free, biologically active androgens and oestradiol.
   **B** **False.**
   **C** **False** – See 11.15D.
   **D** **True** – Raised androgens – testosterone/androstendione from ovarian hypersecretion.

## 11.24 Answers

   **A** **False** – Weight not significantly altered by metformin treatment.
   **B** **False.**
   **C** **False.**
   **D** **False** – Fasting insulin significantly reduced.

## 11.25 Answers

   **A** **True** – Blood pressure – both systolic and diastolic, significantly reduced with metformin compared to placebo.
   **B** **False** – Total cholesterol unchanged but LDL cholesterol significantly reduced. HDL cholesterol and triglycerides unaffected.
   **C** **True** – GI side effects more common with metformin, particularly nausea and vomiting.
   **D** **False.**

## 11.26 Answers

   **A** **True.**
   **B** **False** – SHBG levels not affected.
   **C** **True.**
   **D** **False** – Does not affect long-term risk of NIDDM.

   Note: See 11.19.

   • Laparoscopic ovarian drilling is free of the risks of multiple pregnancy and it does not require ultrasound follicular tracking. As women require test for tubal patency prior to ovulation induction, it may be appropriate to perform ovarian drilling at the same time.

## 11.27 Answers

   **A** **True** – Women with PCOS are at increased risk of adult onset diabetes mellitus – 40% risk of NIDDM by the age of 40 years with truncal obesity and a strong family history of NIDDM being additional risk factors. Offer yearly screening.
   **B** **True** – Mortality from cardiovascular disease is not significantly increased in women with PCOS although they have abnormal lipid profiles. Offer measurement of fasting lipids as early detection of abnormal levels might prompt dietary change and exercise.
   **C** **False** – Metformin decreases insulin resistance but has not been shown to alter the long-term risk of NIDDM.
   **D** **False.**

## 11.28 Answers

**A** **False** – The adrenal gland produces mainly dehydroepiandrosterone sulphate (DHEA-S) with androstendione (equal production with ovaries) and DHEA being produced to a lesser extent. The normal adrenal gland produces little testosterone.

**B** **False** – Main ovarian androgen is testosterone. Ovary also produces androstendione and DHEA.

**C** **True** – Androstendione and DHEA do not have androgenic activity but are converted to testosterone in peripheral tissues.

**D** **True.**

## 11.29 Answers

**A** **True** – 85% of testosterone is bound to sex hormone-binding globulin and is metabolically inactive.

**B** **False** – 10–15% bound to albumin and 1–2% free – free and albumin-bound testosterone are biologically active.

**C** **True** – Testosterone is converted to the biologically active dihydrotestosterone by 5-alpha-reductase. Increased activity of this enzyme may result in the manifestations of androgen excess.

**D** **True.**

Note:

• Two-thirds of daily female testosterone production is of ovarian origin (total = 0.35 mg/day of which 0.1 mg is from direct ovarian production; 0.2 mg from peripheral conversion of androstendione; 0.05 mg from peripheral conversion of DHEA).

## 11.30 Answers

**A** **True.**

**B** **True.**

**C** **True.**

**D** **False.**

Note: Ovarian hyperandrogenaemia:

• Polycystic ovary syndrome, stromal hyperthecosis, ovarian tumours (Sertoli–Leydig cell tumours, Hilus cell tumours, luteomas).

## 11.31 Answers

**A** **True.**

**B** **False.**

**C** **False** – Hirsutism would take several months to resolve after excision of an androgen-secreting tumour.

**D** **False.**

Note:

• Rapidly progressive hirsutism and virilization are suggestive of an androgen-producing tumour of the ovary (Sertoli–Leydig cell tumours, Hilus cell tumours, luteoma) or adrenal cortex.

### 11.32 Answers

**A** True.
**B** False.
**C** False.
**D** True.

Note: Drugs associated with hirsutism:
- Exogenous/iatrogenic androgens – testosterone, anabolic steroids, androgenic progestogens, danazol.
- Phenytoin, cortisone, minoxidil, diazoxide, cyclosporine A – alter the texture and extent of hair growth. The pattern is non-androgenic and is referred to as hypertrichosis.

### 11.33 Answers

**A** **False** – Oral contraceptive pill – suppresses LH production and ovarian androgen synthesis and increases SHBG production, and progesterone inhibits 5-alpha-reductase activity.
**B** **True.**
**C** **True** – Medroxyprogesterone acetate – used in women in whom the COCP is contraindicated – inhibits LH production and ovarian steroidogenesis.
**D** **True** – Progesterone inhibits 5-alpha-reductase activity.

### 11.34 Answers

**A** **False** – Spironolactone is an antiandrogen and aldosterone antagonist. Monitor BP and electrolytes in the first few weeks of treatment – hypotension and hyperkalaemia are side effects.
**B** **False** – Flutamide is a non-steroidal antiandrogen. Hepatotoxicity is a rare side effect – check LFTs.
**C** **False** – Finasteride is a 5-alpha-reductase inhibitor – effective contraception required as can emasculate male fetus.
**D** **True** – Cyproterone acetate is an antiandrogenic progestogen.

### 11.35 Answers

**A** **False** – Teratogenic retinoic acid derivative.
**B** **False** – Teratogenic (emasculates a male fetus).
**C** **False** – Teratogenic retinoic acid derivative.
**D** **True** – Topical benzoyl peroxide is not teratogenic.

## 11.36 Answers

**A** True.
**B** True.
**C** True.
**D** False.

Note: Side effects of clomiphene:

- Visual disturbance – withdraw.
- OHSS – rare.
- Hot flushes, headache, depression, insomnia, convulsions and dizziness.
- Breast tenderness, intermenstrual bleeding, menorrhagia.
- Nausea, vomiting, abdominal discomfort.
- Hair loss.

## 11.37 Answers

**A** **True** – Side effects of cyproterone: fatigue, SOB, hepatotoxicity including jaundice.
**B** **True.**
**C** **True** – Side effects of finasteride: breast tenderness, hypersensitivity reactions, decreased libido.
**D** **True** – Side effects of tamoxifen: hot flushes, abnormal vaginal bleeding, GI disturbance, headache, visual disturbance, VTE, altered liver enzymes.

## 11.38 Answers

**A** True.
**B** True.
**C** False – Androgen insensitivity causes *primary* amenorrhoea.
**D** True.

Note: Causes of secondary amenorrhoea:

- Uterine causes – Asherman's syndrome, cervical stenosis.
- Ovarian causes – PCOS, premature ovarian failure.
- Pituitary causes – hyperprolactinaemia, Sheehan's syndrome, hypothalamic–pituitary damage: tumours including craniopharingiomas, head injury, sarcoidosis, TB.
- Hypothalamic causes – weight loss, anorexia nervosa, exercise, chronic illness, psychological stress.
- Other endocrine disorders – thyroid disease/Cushing's syndrome.

## 11.39 Answers

**A** True.
**B** False – Produced by anterior pituitary lactotrophs, decidua and endometrium.
**C** True.
**D** True.

Note:

- Circulates unbound to serum proteins with a half-life ~20 min.
- Major factor controlling pituitary prolactin secretion is dopamine, produced by the hypothalamus – inhibits pituitary prolactin secretion.

### 11.40 Answers

**A** **True** – Serum prolactin is increased by nipple/breast stimulation, exercise, stress, sleep. Commonest cause of slightly elevated serum prolactin is stress.

**B** **True.**

**C** **False** – Prolactin-secreting *macro*adenomas are associated with a markedly elevated prolactin level.

**D** **True** – Women with PCOS may have mildly elevated prolactin levels.

### 11.41 Answers

**A** **True.**

**B** **True.**

**C** **False** – L-dopa is a dopamine agonist and would inhibit prolactin release.

**D** **True.**

Note: Drugs associated with hyperprolactinaemia:

- Psychotrophic agents – diazepam, phenothiazines, tricyclic antidepressants, opiates, haloperidol.
- Antihypertensives – methyldopa, reserpine, propranolol.
- Hormones – oestrogen, COCP, TRH.
- Antiemetics – metoclopramide, sulpiride.

### 11.42 Answers

**A** **True.**

**B** **True.**

**C** **True.**

**D** **False** – Anorexia nervosa is not associated with hyperprolactinaemia.

Note:

- Causes of hyperprolactinaemia: chronic renal disease, chronic breast nerve stimulation such as that associated with thoracic surgery, herpes zoster and chest trauma.

### 11.43 Answers

**A** **True** – Carbegolline is a long-acting dopamine agonist with a better side-effect profile compared to bromocriptine.

**B** **True.**

**C** **False** – Prolactin levels fall within a few days of therapy and a reduction in tumour volume occurs within 6 weeks. Interpretation of serum prolactin levels in pregnancy is difficult.

**D** **False** – In women with microadenomas, risk of symptoms in pregnancy is 2–5%.

### 11.44 Answers

A **False** – Microadenomas are <10 mm in diameter; macroadenomas are >10 mm diameter.
B **True** – Macroadenomas – 15–33% risk of developing symptoms in pregnancy.
C **False** – Antenatal tumour enlargement should be treated with bromocriptine in the first instance.
D **True** – ACTH +TSH should be assessed – large tumours may interfere with other pituitary functions.

### 11.45 Answers

A **False** – Tumour enlargement causes bitemporal hemianopia.
B **True.**
C **False** – Bromocriptine should be continued if for a macroadenoma.
D **False** – Serum prolactin levels are difficult to interpret in pregnancy but markedly elevated levels may indicate tumour growth.

### 11.46 Answers

A **True.**
B **True.**
C **True.**
D **False.**

Note:

- Side effects of bromocriptine: nausea, vomiting, headache, postural hypotension, constipation, dizziness, drowsiness, Raynaud's phenomenon, psychiatric symptoms, especially aggression, pleural effusion, retroperitomeal fibrosis reported.
- Commence treatment with small dose taken at night with food to minimize side effects.

### 11.47 Answers

A **False.**
B **False.**
C **False.**
D **False.**

## 11.48 Answers

**A** False.
**B** False – Occurs in 3–6% (moderate) or 0.3–0.5% (severe) of stimulated cycles.
**C** True.
**D** False – I.v. albumin may be used to correct volume depletion.

Note:

- Risk factors for OHSS: young age, low body weight, PCOS, high dose of gonadotrophins (rare with oral ovulation induction); large number of oocytes retrieved, high oestradiol levels on the day of HCG administration, pregnancy.
- Complications: hypoalbuminaemia – the ascites fluid is an exudate; electrolyte imbalance – hyponatraemia with hyperkalaemic acidosis; increased thrombogenesis – haemoconcentration and immobility. Arterial, venous and intracerebral thrombosis occurs; cardiorespiratory failure – effusions, ascites and ARDS; pre-renal failure and multiple organ failure; ovarian torsion.
- Diuretics are relatively contraindicated as intravascular volume is reduced.

## 11.49 Answers

**A** False.
**B** False.
**C** False.
**D** True.

Note:

- Males affected (1 in 10 000). Presents at puberty. Normal life-span.
- Reduced or complete absence of the sense of smell (anosmia), underdeveloped genitalia, infertility and lack of secondary sexual characteristics, gynaecomastia, short fourth metacarpal bone. Anosmia is caused by the absence of the olfactory bulbs.
- Hypothalamus is also affected – reduced or absent GnRH, with hypogonadotrophic hypogonadism.
- Ears: serous otitis media is more common. The auricles may be posteriorly rotated as a result of lymphoedema. Hearing loss, due to otosclerosis, is common in adults.
- Gastrointestinal bleeding – due to intestinal vascular malformations. Increased incidence of Crohn's disease and ulcerative colitis.
- Hip dislocation – increased risk.

## 11.50 Answers

**A** True – Autoimmune diseases such as Addison's disease, thyroid disease and diabetes mellitus are associated with premature ovarian failure. In addition, any severe endocrine disorder can cause amenorrhoea.
**B** True – The female with Down syndrome has ovaries containing a reduced number of small follicles, which have a greatly increased rate of atresia.
**C** True – Bulimia and anorexia nervosa are associated with secondary amenorrhoea.
**D** False – Androgen insensitivity syndrome is associated with *primary* amenorrhoea.

### 11.51 Answers

**A** **False** – Clinically indistinguishable from resistant ovary syndrome but ovarian biopsy is not clinically indicated.
**B** **False.**
**C** **False** – Associated with increased risk of cardiovascular disease and osteoporosis but not ovarian cancer.
**D** **True.**

### 11.52 Answers

**A** **False** – Autoimmune disorder in some cases and associated with increased risk of other autoimmune diseases such as thyroid disease and pernicious anaemia.
**B** **False** – Genetic aetiology in up to 40% of cases. Karyotypic abnormalities – commonest being 45,X and 47,XXY followed by mosaiciams and structural abnormalities of sex chromosomes. More common in families with fragile X syndrome.
**C** **True** – See 11.51A.
**D** **False.**

Note:
- Ovarian failure before the age of 40 years.
- Incidence ~1% and 0.1% between the ages of 15 and 29 years.
- Prevalence 10–28% in women with primary amenorrhoea.
- Spontaneous ovulation may occur, therefore ovarian failure is not permanent.
- Aetiology is unknown in most cases. Aetiological factors: autoimmune disorder, genetic, infections – mumps, irradiation/chemotherapy.

# 12. Surgical practice: Questions

**12.1** With regards to suture material:

A Braided sutures handle and knot easier than monofilament sutures.

B Monofilament sutures are less likely to lead to long-term infection compared to braided sutures.

C Catgut is made from the intestines of sheep or cattle.

D Chromic catgut causes more tissue reaction compared to plain catgut.

**12.2** With regards to suture material:

A Catgut is absorbed by hydrolysis.

B Chromic catgut is catgut coated with potassium dichromate to hasten its breakdown.

C Plain catgut loses its tensile strength in about 3 days.

D Chromic catgut loses its tensile strength in about 6 weeks.

**12.3** With regards to suture material:

A Dexon is polyglycolic acid.

B Dexon loses 50% of its tensile strength in 20 days.

C Dexon is completely absorbed within 60 days.

D Vicryl is polydioxanone.

**12.4** With regards to suture material:

A Prolene is a braided suture.

B Prolene is the most permanent non-absorbable suture.

C Ethibond and mersilene are braided sutures made of polyester.

D A 2/0 (00) suture has a wider diameter than a 0 suture.

**12.5** Postoperative pyrexia:

A Occurring on days 0–2 is most likely due to sepsis.

B Occurring on days 0–2 may be due to atelectasis.

C Is a sign of venous thromboembolism.

D Occurring during blood transfusion – transfusion should always be discontinued.

12.6 Tachycardia occurring within 12 hours after hysterectomy may be due to:

A Sepsis.
B Dehydration.
C Poor pain control.
D Excessive intraoperative blood loss.

12.7 Antibiotic prophylaxis in abdominal surgery:

A Is most effective if administered within the 2 hours prior to abdominal incision.
B Reduce the risk of postoperative febrile morbidity.
C Significantly reduces the length of inpatient admission.
D Rectal metronidazole is less effective but cheaper than intravenous metronidazole.

12.8 Wound infection following caesarean section:

A Is more common after emergency compared to elective operations.
B Occurs less commonly in women with intact membranes compared to those with ruptured membranes.
C Occurs in about 1% of patients.
D Antibiotic prophylaxis should be given before the baby is delivered.

12.9 Closure of the peritoneum during caesarean section is associated with:

A Shorter hospital stay.
B Increased requirement for analgesia.
C Increased febrile morbidity.
D Delayed resolution of postoperative ileus.

12.10 The following are indications for therapeutic oophorectomy at the time of hysterectomy:

A Chronic pelvic pain.
B Severe endometriosis.
C Severe pre-menstrual syndrome.
D Strong family history of ovarian cancer.

**12.11** The following groups of women are at increased risk of venous thromboembolism (VTE) following gynaecological surgery:

A Women on the combined oral contraceptive pill.
B Women on HRT.
C Body mass index <25.
D Women undergoing surgery for vulval cancer.

**12.12** The ureter:

A Lies inferior to the uterine artery.
B Lies superior to the cardinal ligament.
C Lies 5 cm lateral to the angle of the vagina.
D Can be protected by carefully reflecting the bladder during hysterectomy.

**12.13** A third-degree tear:

A Is more common with a midline episiotomy.
B Should be repaired under general anaesthesia.
C Should have the anal sphincter repaired before the vaginal skin.
D The anal sphincter should be repaired using vicryl rapide.

**12.14** With respect to the management of abdominal pain:

A Urgent surgical intervention is indicated in a patient who presents with an appendicular mass.
B A normal white cell count does not exclude the diagnosis of appendicitis.
C Laparotomy and surgical excision is appropriate treatment in a 25-year-old woman who is found to have severe endometriosis at laparoscopy.

**12.15** A 30-year-old woman presents with abdominal pain at 24 weeks' gestation:

A Quiescent ulcerative colitis is likely to relapse during pregnancy.
B An ultrasound scan can exclude placental abruption.
C If appendicitis is suspected, laparoscopy is indicated.
D Acute salpingitis is a likely cause of pain localized to the right iliac fossa.

**12.16** Compared to general anaesthesia, regional anaesthesia used during major surgery is associated with:

A An increased blood loss.

B An increased risk of deep venous thrombosis.

C Better postoperative pain control.

D Lower risk of postoperative nausea.

**12.17** Administration of epidural analgesia in early labour is associated with:

A An increased risk of caesarean section.

B Prolongation of the first stage of labour compared to use of intramuscular opioids.

C Prolongation of the second stage of labour compared to use of intramuscular opioids.

D Lower intrapartum pain scores compared to use of intramuscular opioids.

**12.18** With respect to continuous lumbar epidural analgesia:

A The procedure must be abandoned if a spinal tap occurs during administration.

B It is contraindicated in suspected IUGR.

C Respiratory arrest is a recognized complication.

D It should not be administered during the second stage of labour.

**12.19** With respect to continuous lumbar epidural analgesia:

A Leakage of cerebrospinal fluid is a recognized cause of headache.

B It is contraindicated in women with a past history of DVT.

C Hypertension treated with labetalol is a recognized contraindication.

D There is an increased risk of PPH.

# Answers

## 12.1 Answers

**A** **True** – Braided sutures: strands are plaited, making the sutures very flexible, easy to handle and knot, knots secure. Monofilament sutures are one strand, less flexible, more slippery, more difficult to handle and knot. Knots need more throws to be secure.

**B** **True** – The interstices of the yarn of braided sutures may provide a nidus for microbes.

**C** **True** – Catgut is strands of collagen from sheep/cow intestine. Now phased out in the UK.

**D** **False** – Chromic catgut is coated in potassium dichromate and causes less inflammation.

## 12.2 Answers

**A** **False** – Catgut is absorbed by proteases.

**B** **False.**

**C** **True** – Plain catgut loses tensile strength in ~5 days.

**D** **False** – Chromic catgut loses tensile strength in 14–21 days.

## 12.3 Answers

**A** **True.**

**B** **True** – Dexon is braided and loses 50% of its tensile strength in 20 days.

**C** **False** – Dexon is absorbed by hydrolysis in 100–120 days.

**D** **False** – Vicryl is polygalactin. It is braided and causes minimal tissue reaction, loses 60% of tensile strength in 20 days, and is absorbed by hydrolysis at 60–90 days.

## 12.4 Answers

**A** **False** – Prolene (polypropylene) is a monofilament; minimal tissue reaction, most permanent non-absorbable suture, suitable for subcuticular sutures.

**B** **True.**

**C** **True** – Mersilene is a polyester fibre; braided, little tissue reaction. Ethibond is a braided polyester coated with surgical lubricant, travels smoothly through tissue and knots securely.

**D** **False** – Thickness or calibre is conventionally described as 'number 1', 'number 2' – increasing thickness, or '0', '2/0' – decreasing thickness.

## 12.5 Answers

**A False** – Unlikely to be due to sepsis, although streptococcal and clostridial infections may present with early post-op fever.

**B True.**

**C True.**

**D False** – If a low-grade transfusion reaction occurs, slow rate of transfusion but do not necessarily discontinue transfusion.

Note: Causes of post-op pyrexia:

- Early (<24 hours): atelectasis, transfusion reaction, VTE, peritoneal soiling – occult bowel injury/anastomotic leak, urinoma – occult ureteric or bladder injury, unexplained fever – may be due to drugs.
- Late (>36 hours): All causes of early post-op pyrexia, infections – UTI, pneumonia, wound infection, pelvic collection (blood or pus), haematoma, thrombophlebitis.

## 12.6 Answers

**A False** – Sepsis is unlikely to present within the first 12 hours post-op.

**B True.**

**C True.**

**D True.**

Note:

- Causes of early post-op tachycardia: blood loss, dehydration, pain, VTE, myocardial infarction.

## 12.7 Answers

**A True** – Most effective if administered in the 2 hours preceding abdominal incision – 0.6% wound infection rate compared to 3.8% if >2 hours before incision, and 1.4% if up to 3 hours after incision.

**B True** – Associated with ~30% reduction in the risk of post-op febrile morbidity.

**C False** – Length of hospital stay is not significantly reduced.

**D False** – Rectal metronidazole is as effective as i.v. regimen in reducing febrile morbidity and is cheaper.

## 12.8 Answers

**A True** – Rates ~4.7% after elective and up to 24% after emergency C/S.

**B True** – More common in the presence of PROM, anaemia, cord prolapse, meconium-stained liquor.

**C False.**

**D False** – Prophylactic antibiotics should be administered after the fetus has been delivered and the cord clamped. Poly-microbial for *Staph. aureus*, *E. coli*, Bacteroides, beta-haemolytic strep.

## 12.9 Answers

A **False** – Non-closure is associated with shorter operating time (parietal), shorter hospital stay.

B **True** – Non-closure is associated with lower use of analgesia (parietal peritoneum).

C **True** – Non-closure is associated with lower risk of post-op febrile and infectious morbidity (visceral).

D **True** – Non-closure is associated with a quicker return of bowel activity.

Note:
- Peritoneal closure is associated with an increased incidence of bladder adhesions and is not cost-effective.

## 12.10 Answers

A **True** – In women with chronic pelvic pain, endometriosis or severe PMS, oophorectomy is potentially therapeutic.

B **True.**

C **True.**

D **False** – In women with a family history of ovarian cancer, breast cancer or perimenopausal women, oophorectomy is prophylactic.

Note:
- Oophorectomy may be prophylactic or therapeutic.

## 12.11 Answers

A **True** – COCP is associated with increased risk of VTE and should be stopped at least 6 weeks before major elective surgery.

B **True** – HRT is associated with increased risk of VTE but should not necessarily be stopped before major elective surgery; it should be considered during risk assessment.

C **False** – BMI >30.

D **True.**

Note: Risk factors for VTE:
- Increasing age (>35).
- Immobility.
- Obesity.
- Previous VTE.
- Thrombophilia.
- Dehydration.
- Malignancy.
- Blood group (Group O protective).
- Medical disorders – congestive cardiac failure, nephrotic syndrome, polycythaemia vera, essential thrombocythaemia.
- Inflammatory disorders (bowel disease, UTIs).
- Excessive blood loss.
- COCP and HRT.

## 12.12 Answers

**A** True.

**B** True.

**C** False.

**D** True – The ureter is at risk of injury during gynaecological surgery at four points: the pelvic brim (may be confused with the infundibulo-pelvic ligament), lateral to the ovarian fossa, the ureteric tunnel beneath the uterine artery and anterior to the vagina where it runs into the bladder. Adequate reflection of the bladder minimizes the risk of distal ureteric injury.

Note: The ureter in the pelvis:

- Enters the pelvis anterior to the bifurcation of the common iliac artery.
- Descends on the pelvic side-wall medial to the branches of the internal iliac artery and lateral to the ovarian fossa.
- Runs lateral to the utero-sacral ligament , superior to the cardinal ligament.
- Runs inferior to the uterine artery 1–1.5 cm lateral to the cervix and the vagina.

## 12.13 Answers

**A** True – Midline episiotomy increases the risk of third-degree tears.

**B** False – Repair should be undertaken in the operating theatre with good lighting and appropriate analgesia/anaesthesia.

**C** True.

**D** False.

Note: Repair of third- and fourth-degree lacerations:

- The full extent of the injury should be ascertained.
- The anal epithelium should be repaired with 3-0 polygalactin sutures (Vicryl).
- The internal anal sphincter should be identified and repaired using interrupted or mattress 3-0 polydioxanone (PDS).
- The external anal sphincter should be repaired using 2-0 PDS – an end-to-end or overlapping technique may be used.
- The vaginal epithelium is then closed using a loose continuous non-locking stitch with rapid absorbable 2-0 polygalactin.
- The perineal body should be re-constructed to support the sphincter repair using interrupted 2-0 polygalactin.
- The perineal skin is closed using subcuticular 2-0 rapid absorbable polygalactin.

## 12.14 Answers

**A** True – Suspected appendicular mass should be managed by resuscitation and urgent appendectomy/laparotomy.

**B** True – Normal white cell count/CRP/temperature do not exclude a diagnosis of appendicitis.

**C** False – Severe endometriosis is best managed surgically by laser laparoscopy in a tertiary centre.

## 12.15 Answers

**A** **False** – Autoimmune diseases in remission are less likely to relapse antenatally. Increased risk of relapse post-partum.

**B** **False** – Placental abruption is a clinical diagnosis and cannot be excluded by ultrasound scan.

**C** **False** – Suspected appendicitis in pregnancy should be managed by open appendectomy or laparotomy.

**D** **False** – Acute salpingitis is extremely rare in a woman with an ongoing pregnancy.

## 12.16 Answers

**A** **False** – Regional anaesthesia is associated with reduced blood loss due to lower arterial and venous pressures.

**B** **False** – Reduced rates of deep venous thrombosis – improved blood flow through the legs secondary to sympathectomy-induced vasodilation and also reduced perioperative hypercoagulability that occurs because of the surgical stress response.

**C** **True** – Better pain control – can block or reduce pain from several hours to several days, depending on the technique used. Better pain control has the potential to allow for earlier mobilization and discharge.

**D** **True** – Regional anaesthesia avoids common adverse effects of general anesthesia – nausea, sore throat, alteration of mental status and cognitive dysfunction.

Note:
* Regional anaesthesia allows patient involvement, which is especially relevant to child-birth.

## 12.17 Answers

**A** **False.**
**B** **False.**
**C** **False.**
**D** **True.**

Note: Epidural and outcome of labour (Wong CA et al *N Engl J Med* 2005;**352**:655–665):
* Rate of C/S was not significantly different between the groups (17.8% after intrathecal analgesia vs 20.7% after systemic analgesia).
* The median time from the initiation of analgesia to complete dilatation was significantly shorter after intrathecal analgesia than after systemic analgesia (295 minutes vs 385 minutes, P<0.001).
* The time to vaginal delivery was significantly shorter after intrathecal analgesia than after systemic analgesia (398 minutes vs 479 minutes, P<0.001).
* Pain scores after the first intervention were significantly lower after intrathecal analgesia than after systemic analgesia (2 vs 6 on a 0–10 scale, P<0.001).
* The incidence of 1-minute Apgar scores below 7 was significantly higher after systemic analgesia (24.0% vs 16.7%, P=0.01).

### 12.18 Answers

    **A** **False** – Spinal tap – if analgesia is intended for operative intervention, proceed with subarachnoid block (spinal) using bupivacaine + opioid. If for labour, consider administering spinal and inserting epidural at another level.

    **B** **False** – Contraindications to epidural analgesia: patient refusal, active maternal haemorrhage, maternal septicaemia or untreated febrile illness, infection at or near needle insertion site, maternal coagulopathy, allergy to local anaesthetic/opiates.

    **C** **True** – Complications include total spinal anaesthesia – secondary to unintentional subarachnoid injection of local anaesthetic. This is an emergency with altered consciousness, hypotension, bradycardia, respiratory depression/arrest.

    **D** **False** – May be administered during second stage of labour.

### 12.19 Answers

    **A** **True** – Delayed complications include postdural puncture headache – typically postural, and results from leakage of CSF, with a decrease in intracranial pressure and compensatory cerebral vasodilation. There is also traction on pain-sensitive intracranial structures.

    **B** **False** – See 12.18B.

    **C** **False** – See 12.18B.

    **D** **False**.

# 13. Neonatology and epidemiology: Questions

**13.1** With respect to brachial plexus injury:

A Erb's palsy is associated with injury to C5/6 nerve roots.
B Klumpke's palsy is associated with C8–T1 injury.
C Klumpke's palsy is associated with Horner's syndrome.
D Physiotherapy is the main mode of treatment.

**13.2** With regard to intra/extracranial haemorrhage

A Cephalohaematomas are uncommon after normal deliveries.
B Cephalohaematomas cross the midline.
C Subaponeurotic haemorrhage crosses the midline.
D Subaponeurotic haemorrhage may be associated with neonatal shock.

**13.3** With regard to intra/extracranial haemorrhage:

A Subaponeurotic haemorrhage carries a 15–20% mortality.
B Subarachnoid haemorrhage generally carries a poor prognosis.
C Tentorial tears are associated with vaginal breech deliveries.
D Intraventricular haemorrhage may be an incidental finding in 2% of normal term babies.

**13.4** In the use of vitamin K to prevent haemorrhagic disease of the newborn:

A Breastfed babies given intramuscular vitamin K at birth do not require further supplementation.
B Oral vitamin K given for the first month of life is as effective as intramuscular vitamin K.
C Vitamin K supplementation should be continued for 3 months in formula-fed infants.
D Breastfed babies require oral vitamin K supplementation until weaned.

**13.5** The following groups of babies are at increased risk of haemorrhagic disease of the newborn:

A Premature babies.
B Macrosomic babies.
C Babies born to women on anticonvulsants.
D Babies delivered by forceps.

**13.6** Regarding antenatal and neonatal thyroid disease:

A Maternal thyroxine and TSH do not cross the placenta in significant amounts.
B Carbimazole does not cross the placenta.
C In maternal Graves' disease, IgM antibodies can cross the placenta and cause neonatal thyrotoxicosis.
D Neonatal hypothyroidism may present with jaundice, poor feeding, hypotonia and poor temperature control.

**13.7** Regarding antenatal and neonatal thyroid disease:

A Transient neonatal hypothyroidism may be caused by thyroid agenesis.
B Maternal Graves' disease carries a 2% risk of neonatal hyperthyroidism.
C Carbimazole and propylthiouracil both suppress maternal production of thyroid-stimulating antibodies.
D In a woman with a previous history of Graves' disease who is euthyroid in pregnancy there is no risk of neonatal thyroid disease.

**13.8** Congenital hypothyroidism:

A Maternal antithyroid therapy is the commonest cause.
B Most cases are transient and do not require any treatment.
C Screening is based on detecting low neonatal levels of T3 and T4.
D Screening should be performed in the first 48 hours of life.

**13.9** The Guthrie test:

A Screens for hypothyroidism.
B Should be undertaken within 24 h of birth.
C May be affected by antibiotic treatment.
D Screens for phenylketonuria.

**13.10** The following conditions cause unconjugated neonatal hyperbilirubinaemia:

A Haemolysis.
B Cystic fibrosis.
C Polycythaemia.
D Intrauterine infection.

**13.11** The following conditions cause unconjugated neonatal hyperbilirubinaemia:

A Pyloric stenosis.
B Biliary atresia.
C Hypothyroidism.
D Cephalohaematoma.

**13.12** With regards to jaundice in the term neonate:

A About 50% of healthy breastfed infants become jaundiced.
B Breastfeeding should be temporarily discontinued if jaundice develops.
C Physiological jaundice occurs in days 7–10 of life.
D Babies with physiological jaundice may show signs of systemic illness.

**13.13** Excess urobilinogen in the urine is a recognized feature of:

A Cholestatic jaundice of pregnancy.
B Hereditary spherocytosis.
C Sickle cell disease.
D Acute fatty liver of pregnancy.

**13.14** A 5-year-old boy is thought to have suffered intrapartum asphyxia. The following would support the diagnosis:

A Cardiotocographic evidence of fetal distress.
B Antenatal evidence of IUGR.
C Cord pH of 7.25.
D Low Apgar scores at 1 minute.

**13.15** The following are components of the Apgar score:

A Respiratory rate.
B Heart rate.
C Colour.
D Response to stimulation.

**13.16** The following are recognized complications of babies born to diabetic mothers:

A Brachial plexus injury.
B Neonatal hyperglycaemia.
C Transient tachypnoea of the newborn.
D Jaundice.

**13.17** The following are complications of babies born to diabetic mothers:

A Anaemia.
B Poor suckling and swallowing.
C Cardiomyopathy.
D Thrombocytopenia.

**13.18** Facial nerve palsy:

A Is associated with forceps delivery.
B Does not occur following normal vaginal delivery.
C Is associated with ventouse delivery.
D The majority require reconstructive surgery.

**13.19** During development of the genital tract and gonads:

A The Y chromosome has a testis-determining factor on its long arm (Yq).
B The sex cords become canalized to form seminiferous tubules during the seventh month of development.
C The upper two-thirds of the vagina is derived from the Müllerian tubercle.
D Complete canalization of the vagina does not occur until after delivery.

**13.20** With respect to sexual development:

A Two functional X chromosomes are essential for normal ovarian development.
B In the absence of a Y chromosome the external genitalia develops a female phenotype.
C Testosterone is essential for development of the male phenotype.
D The ovaries are essential for normal phenotypic female development.

**13.21** Congenital uterine anomalies are typically associated with the following:

A Renal tract anomalies.
B Androgen insensitivity syndrome.
C Malpresentation.
D Placenta previa.

**13.22** With respect to congenital adrenal hyperplasia:

A Only female fetuses are affected.
B 21-hydroxylase deficiency is the commonest enzyme abnormality.
C Salt-losing syndrome is characterized by low plasma potassium.
D Cortisol levels are elevated.

**13.23** Congenital adrenal hyperplasia:

A Is inherited as an X-linked condition.
B May be caused by 11-hydroxylase deficiency.
C Is associated with absent uterus and fallopian tubes and a blind-ending vagina.
D May be caused by 3-beta hydroxysteroid dehydrogenase deficiency.

**13.24** With respect to congenital adrenal hyperplasia:

A Prenatal diagnosis is possible.
B Androstendione levels are increased.
C Genetically male infants have ambiguous genitalia at birth.
D Corticosteroid replacement is required.

**13.25** Necrotizing enterocolitis is characterized by:

A Blood in the stool.
B Abdominal distension.
C Bile-stained vomit.
D An association with preterm delivery.

**13.26** Necrotizing enterocolitis is characterized by:

A An association with severe IUGR.
B A higher incidence in breast- than bottle-fed babies.
C An association with neonatal respiratory distress.
D Intramural gas on abdominal X-ray.

**13.27** Necrotizing enterocolitis is characterized by:

A Free intraperitoneal gas on abdominal X-ray.
B A higher incidence in neonates who have not received oral feeding.
C Mortality rates of about 1%.
D A 30% risk of ischaemic colonic strictures in survivors.

**13.28** Puerperal mastitis:

A Typically presents with an inflamed tender area of breast surrounding the nipple.
B May require culture of breast milk if not responding to treatment.
C If recurrent, may indicate the presence of ductal carcinoma.
D Should be treated with clindamycin in a woman with severe penicillin allergy.

**13.29** In a woman with puerperal mastitis:

A Suckling should be discouraged on the affected breast.
B Group A streptococci are the commonest causative organisms.
C Penicillinase-resistant antibiotics should be administered.
D Cessation of breastfeeding results in symptomatic improvement.

**13.30** Compared to bottle-feeding, breastfeeding is associated with:

A A lower risk of sudden infant death syndrome.
B A lower risk of atopic eczema.
C A higher risk of necrotizing enterocolitis.
D A higher risk of diarrhoea.

**13.31** Compared to bottle-feeding, breastfeeding is associated with:

A A lower risk of pneumonia.
B A lower risk of inflammatory bowel disease.
C A higher risk of requiring tonsillectomy.
D A lower risk of constipation.

**13.32** Congenital dislocation of the hip (developmental dysplasia of the hip):

A Is more common in girls than in boys.
B Is more likely after a vaginal breech delivery than after C/S.
C Affects 1% of neonates.
D Can be excluded by hip examination undertaken within 48 hours of delivery.

**13.33** Developmental dysplasia of the hip (congenital dislocation of the hip):

A Is more common in girls than in boys.
B Is bilateral in over 50% of cases.
C Is associated with breech presentation at term.
D Is more common in the presence of polyhydramnios.

**13.34** Developmental dysplasia of the hip (congenital dislocation of the hip):

A Is diagnosed by the presence of clicky hips in the neonatal period.
B Is more common in first-born children.
C Is more common in multiple pregnancy.
D Is more common in the presence of oligohydramnios.

**13.35** Developmental dysplasia of the hip (congenital dislocation of the hip):

A Is treated initially by closed reduction under general anaesthesia.
B Resolves spontaneously in about 5% of cases.
C Affects the right hip more often than the left.
D Is screened for using the Barlow and Ortolani tests.

**13.36** A healthy normotensive 42-year-old woman is pregnant for the first time. Compared to a healthy 25-year-old woman, she is:

A Significantly more likely to have higher fasting blood glucose concentrations.
B More likely to have a molar pregnancy.
C Three times more likely to have an ectopic pregnancy.
D Less likely to have a baby with a neural tube defect.

**13.37** In a pregnant woman over the age of 35 years, there is:

A An increased risk of multiple pregnancy.
B An increased risk of hyperthyroidism.
C An increased risk of gestational diabetes.
D An increased risk of hypertension in pregnancy.

**13.38** In a pregnant woman over the age of 35 years, there is:

A  A decreased risk of ectopic pregnancy.
B  A decreased risk of placenta previa.
C  Increased risk of monozygotic twins.
D  Increased risk of trophoblastic disease.

**13.39** In a pregnant woman over the age of 35 years, there is:

A  Increased risk of placental abruption.
B  Increased risk of fatal thromboembolism.
C  A decreased risk of preterm delivery.
D  Increased risk of prolonged second stage of labour.

# Answers

## 13.1 Answers

**A** **True** – Erb–Duchenne palsy is associated with C5/C6 nerve root injury, caused by excessive displacement of the head to the opposite side or depression of the shoulder on the same side.

**B** **True** – Klumpke's palsy is associated with C8/T1. Small muscles of the hand are paralyzed causing claw hand. Sensory loss on medial side of arm.

**C** **True**.

**D** **True** – Treatment is by physiotherapy ± reconstructive surgery.

Note:

- Most babies with brachial plexus injury have near normal function but only ~20% have full neurological recovery. Majority of recovery occurs in the first month.

## 13.2 Answers

**A** **False** – Incidence of cephalohaematoma, 1%.

**B** **False** – Beneath periosteum, swelling does not cross suture lines.

**C** **True** – Subaponeurotic (subgleal) haemorrhage: rare, bleed beneath the aponeurosis, crosses midline.

**D** **True** – Associated with shock/anaemia and neonatal death. Increased incidence with ventouse delivery.

Note:

- Cephalohaematoma is associated with jaundice. May not appear until second day of life and may take several weeks to finally disappear.

## 13.3 Answers

**A** **True**.

**B** **False** – Subarachnoid haemorrhage is from small vessels (usually veins) within the subarachnoid space. Usually silent but may be associated with fits – good prognosis.

**C** **True** – Tentorial tears are thought to occur following sudden decompression of the after-coming head in vaginal breech delivery.

**D** **True** – Germinal matrix/intraventricular haemorrhage occurs in ~2% of normal babies at term. Increased incidence in preterm. Good prognosis if germinal matrix only involved. Poorer outcome if brain parenchyma involved.

### 13.4 Answers

**A** **True** – I mg vitamin K given i.m. at birth is sufficient to prevent HDN. No further supplementation required even if breastfed.

**B** **False** – Oral regimens available – 2 mg at birth.

**C** **False** – Bottle-feed is supplemented with vitamin K and further doses are not required in bottle-fed babies.

**D** **True** – Breastfed babies given oral vitamin K at birth require further oral supplementation – 2 mg at I week and I month of age, and repeated monthly until weaned.

Note:

- Neonates have relative vitamin K deficiency and may suffer haemorrhagic complications which can be fatal. Incidence ~1:10 000 if untreated.

### 13.5 Answers

**A** **True.**

**B** **False.**

**C** **True.**

**D** **True.**

Note:

- Babies at high risk of HDN: preterm, small for gestational age, badly bruised, breech deliveries, operative delivery, maternal anticonvulsant therapy, maternal/neonatal liver disease, admission to SCBU, poor feeding.
- I.m. vitamin K recommended.

### 13.6 Answers

**A** **True** – Thyroxine does not cross the placenta in clinically significant amounts.

**B** **False** – Antithyroid drugs cross the placenta and can cause neonatal hypothyroidism.

**C** **False** – Thyroid-stimulating antibodies are IgG.

**D** **True** – Neonatal hypothyroidism may present with hypotonia, poor feeding and temperature control, jaundice.

### 13.7 Answers

**A** **False** – Thyroid agenesis causes permanent disease requiring long-term treatment.

**B** **True.**

**C** **True** – Antithyroid drugs suppress the production of antithyroid antibodies.

**D** **False** – Risk remains in treated women, even those who are hypothyroid.

## 13.8 Answers

**A** **False** – Incidence 1:4000 deliveries. Causes: thyroid dysgenesis/agenesis (75%), dyshormonogenesis (20%), isoimmune (5%), transient neonatal hypothyroidism (10–20%).

**B** **False** – Untreated causes severe mental impairment (cretinism). Good outcome if early recognition and treatment.

**C** **False** – Screening: TSH assay from heel-prick sample obtained at same time as Guthrie test.

**D** **False.**

## 13.9 Answers

**A** **False** – Screens for phenylketonuria. Bacterial inhibition assay on blood adsorbed onto blotting paper.

**B** **False** – Infant needs to be on an adequate milk diet for 48 hours before testing.

**C** **True** – Antibiotic treatment may confound test.

**D** **True.**

Note: Phenylketonuria (PKU):

- Autosomal recessive, deficiency of phenylalanine hydroxylase.
- Untreated causes neonatal convulsions and subsequent mental impairment and epilepsy, and is associated with eczema.
- Affected children have fair hair/skin with blue eyes – relative melanin deficiency.
- Treat with low phenylalanine/tryptophan diet within 20 days of birth – life-long or at least into adulthood. Good outcome.
- Women with PKU need to have disease adequately controlled before conception – risk of fetal brain damage by transplacental passage of phenylpyruvate products.

## 13.10 Answers

**A** **True.**
**B** **False.**
**C** **True.**
**D** **False.**

## 13.11 Answers

**A** **True.**
**B** **False.**
**C** **True.**
**D** **True.**

Note:

- Increased incidence of unconjugated neonatal hyperbilirubinaemia with prematurity, bruising, instrumental delivery (RCTs show no difference in need for phototherapy between ventouse and forceps delivery), breastfeeding, polycythaemia.
- Causes of conjugated hyperbilirubinaemia: sepsis, biliary atresia, cystic fibrosis, alpha-1-antitrypsin deficiency, choledochal cyst, prolonged TPN, galactosaemia.

### 13.12 Answers

**A** **True** – Physiological: transient rise in serum bilirubin in all neonates, 30–50% of term neonates are jaundiced – unconjugated hyperbilirubinaemia. Caused by high haematocrit, shorter life-span of red cells, immature hepatic enzymes and increased enterohepatic circulation.

**B** **False** – Breastfeeding should be continued.

**C** **False** – Peak concentration of serum bilirubin on day 3, cleared by day 10.

**D** **False.**

### 13.13 Answers

**A** **False.**

**B** **True.**

**C** **True.**

**D** **True.**

Note:

- Both bilirubin and urobilinogen may be detected in urine.
- Partial or complete biliary obstruction or liver damage may cause bilirubinuria. The excreted bilirubin is conjugated.
- Urinary urobilinogen may be increased in hepatocellular diseases, but is not affected by partial biliary obstruction and may be decreased with complete obstruction.
- Haemolysis causes increased conjugation of bilirubin with glucuronic acid in the liver. The conjugated bilirubin is excreted into the bile, where it is metabolized to stercobilinogen and urobilinogen. Some of the urobilinogen re-absorbed from the gastrointestinal tract is subsequently excreted in the urine.
- Increased urobilinogen in urine therefore occurs in: excessive RBC breakdown, re-absorption – a large hematoma, hepatocellular damage.

### 13.14 Answers

**A** **True.**

**B** **False.**

**C** **False** – pH <7.0.

**D** **False.**

Note: Birth asphyxia: The following criteria should be fulfilled before long-term outcome can be attributed to acute intrapartum events:

- Essential criteria: evidence of intrapartum metabolic acidosis in intrapartum fetal, umbilical arterial or very early neonatal sample (pH <7.0, base deficit >12 mmol/L); early onset of severe or moderately severe hypoxic ischaemic encephalopathy in an infant >34 weeks' gestation, cerebral palsy of the spastic quadriplegic or dystonic type.
- Additional criteria: delayed onset of respiration/low Apgar scores (0–6 for longer than 5 minutes); early evidence of multiorgan involvement – in particular renal failure; a sentinel hypoxic event occurring immediately before or during labour; sudden, rapid and sustained deterioration in the fetal heart rate pattern; early imaging evidence of acute cerebral abnormality.

## 13.15 Answers

**A** False.
**B** True.
**C** True.
**D** True.

Note:
- Apgar score: heart rate, respiratory effort, muscle tone, reflex irritability, colour.

## 13.16 Answers

**A** True.
**B** False.
**C** True.
**D** True.

## 13.17 Answers

**A** False.
**B** True.
**C** True.
**D** False.

Note: Neonatal risks of diabetes in pregnancy:
- Macrosomia associated with birth injury, including brachial plexus injury.
- Neonatal hypoglycaemia, hypocalcaemia and hypomagnesaemia.
- Increased risk of respiratory distress and transient tachypnoea.
- Polycythaemia and neonatal jaundice.
- Cardiomyopathy occurs in ~1% of neonates.

## 13.18 Answers

**A** True – Associated with forceps delivery but can be spontaneous (prolonged pressure on sacral promontory).
**B** False.
**C** False.
**D** False – Treat with eye patch + artificial tears.

Note:
- Inability to close eye and lack of lower lip depression on affected side. Usually transient.

## 13.19 Answers

**A** False – Y-chromosome has a testis-determining factor on its short arm (Yp).
**B** False – Testis cords become canalized at puberty, forming seminiferous tubules.
**C** False – Upper third of the vagina develops from the fused Müllerian ducts, lower two-thirds develop from the urogenital sinus.
**D** False – Becomes canalized during the fifth month of development.

### 13.20 Answers

**A** **True** – In the absence of a Y chromosome or in the absence of a gonad, development would be female in nature. However, two functional X chromosomes are required for optimal ovarian development.

**B** **True.**

**C** **True** – Development of the Wolffian duct is under direct influence of testosterone. Development of the external genitalia in the male requires conversion of testosterone to dihydrotestosterone by 5-alpha-reductase.

**D** **False** – In the absence of testosterone, the mesonephric system degenerates in the female – ovaries are not essential for the development of a normal female phenotype.

### 13.21 Answers

**A** **True** – Associated with renal tract and vaginal anomalies (renal ultrasound scan ± IVP).

**B** **False.**

**C** **True** – May cause malpresentation. A rudimentary horn of the uterus may obstruct labour.

**D** **False.**

Note:

- Fusion abnormalities – spectrum from bicornuate uterus, to septate uterus to uterus didelphys.

### 13.22 Answers

**A** **False** – Autosomal recessive condition, males also affected.

**B** **True** – Commonest enzyme defect is 21-hydroxylase deficiency (90% of cases). 11-beta-hydroxylase deficiency and 3-beta-hydroxysteroid dehydrogenase deficiency are less common causes.

**C** **False** – Salt-losing syndrome is characterized by low cortisol.

**D** **False.**

### 13.23 Answers

**A** **False** – See 13.22A.

**B** **True** – See 13.22B.

**C** **False** – Associated with clitoral enlargement; fusion of genital folds; thickening and rugosity of tha labia majora which resemble the scrotum. Uterus, fallopian tubes and vagina are always present although the introitus may be difficult to identify.

**D** **True** – See 13.22B.

## 13.24 Answers

**A** **True** – Offer prenatal diagnosis/genetic counselling in subsequent pregnancy.

**B** **True** – Raised ACTH, 17-hydroxyprogesterone, progesterone, androstendione, testosterone.

**C** **False** – Syndrome may be unrecognized in the male and later presents with precocious puberty.

**D** **True** – Cortisol replacement suppresses ACTH overproduction. Surgical correction of external genitalia.

Note:

- Congenital adrenal hyperplasia is the commonest cause of female intersex; incidence ~1:15 000 live births.
- Salt losing characterized by low $Na^+/Cl^-$ and raised $K^+$.
- Menarche delayed by 2 years, reduced fertility.

## 13.25 Answers

**A** **True** – Usually occurs in the first week of life. Baby is lethargic with vomiting, hypotonia, apnoea. Bloody diarrhoea is a late feature.

**B** **True** – Abdominal examination may show abdominal distension with peritonitis or abdominal mass. Abdominal X-ray may show distended bowel with mucosal oedema, intramural gas, portal venous gas or free intraperitoneal gas. Portal venous gas is a poor prognostic sign.

**C** **False.**

**D** **True** – Associated with: prematurity/PPROM, prolonged labour, hypoxia and respiratory distress, severe IUGR, umbilical artery catheterization.

## 13.26 Answers

**A** **True** – See 13.25D.

**B** **False** – Less common in breastfed neonates.

**C** **True** – See 13.25D.

**D** **True** – See 13.25B.

## 13.27 Answers

**A** **True** – See 13.25B.

**B** **False.**

**C** **False** – Mortality ~ 20% following medical treatment; ~30% if surgery needed.

**D** **True** – 30% risk of ischaemic colonic strictures in survivors.

## 13.28 Answers

**A** **False** – Presents with a tender, hot, red swollen wedge-shaped area of breast with pyrexia (>38°C) and systemic illness. However, a bacterial infection is not necessarily present.

**B** **True** – WHO recommends that breast milk culture should be undertaken if there is no response to antibiotics within 48 hours, if symptoms recur, in hospital-acquired mastitis or in severe/unusual cases.

**C** **True** – Two to three recurrences in the same location requires assessment to exclude underlying mass, inflammatory or ductal carcinoma and resistant bacterial strains.

**D** **True.**

## 13.29 Answers

**A** **False** – See D.

**B** **False** – *Staph. aureus* is commonest causative organism. *E. coli* also detected.

**C** **True** – Penicillinase-resistant antibiotic such as flucloxacillin is first-line antibiotic. Clindamycin if penicillin allergy.

**D** **False** – Most effective initial management strategy is frequent and effective milk removal – encourage more frequent breastfeeding starting with the affected breast.

Note:
• Mastitis affects up to 20% of women in the first 6 months after delivery.

## 13.30 Answers

**A** **True.**
**B** **True.**
**C** **False.**
**D** **False.**

## 13.31  Answers

   **A** True.
   **B** True.
   **C** False.
   **D** True.

Note: Benefits of breastfeeding:

- Ears: fewer ear infections.
- Throat: less likely to require tonsillectomies.
- Respiratory system: fewer and less severe upper respiratory infections, less wheezing, less pneumonia and less influenza.
- Digestive system: less diarrhoea/constipation, fewer gastrointestinal infections. Six months or more of exclusive breastfeeding reduces risk of food allergies. Lower risk of Crohn's disease and ulcerative colitis in adulthood. Lower risk of necrotizing enterocolitis.
- Immune system: better response to immunization.
- Endocrine system: lower risk of IDDM.
- Urinary tract: fewer UTIs.
- Growth: leaner at 1 year of age and less likely to be obese later in life.
- Skin: less allergic eczema.
- CNS: lower risk of bacterial meningitis and sudden infant death syndrome.
- Enhances cognitive development.

## 13.32  Answers

   **A** **True** – Female:male ratio ~ 8:1.
   **B** **False.**
   **C** **False** – Incidence 0.5–1.5% of neonates at birth but only 1–2 per 1000 have persistent hip instability.
   **D** **False.**

## 13.33  Answers

   **A** **True** – Female:male ratio ~ 8:1.
   **B** **False** – Bilateral in 20–40%.
   **C** **True** – Risk factors include: female sex, familial history (6% risk if one previous affected child; 12% if present in a parent), breech presentation; multiple pregnancy, first pregnancy, high birth weight, oligohydramnios and postural and non-postural abnormalities like clubfoot and congenital torticollis. More common in Caucasians.
   **D** **False** – More common in the presence of *oligo*hydramnios.

## 13.34  Answers

   **A** **False** – Hip clicks are benign findings and they are the result of stretching and snapping of the joint capsule and tendons.
   **B** **True** – See 13.33C.
   **C** **True** – See 13.33C.
   **D** **True** – See 13.33C.

### 13.35 Answers

**A** **False** – Most unstable hips in neonates normalize spontaneously within the first 2–4 weeks of birth. Expectant management in the first instance. Splinting may later be required but not appropriate if child is over 6 months old. Closed reduction under GA or open reduction are other options.

**B** **False.**

**C** **False** – Left hip is affected three times more often than the right.

**D** **True** – *Barlow test* determines if a hip is dislocatable. The femur is flexed and adducted while posteriorly directed pressure is applied. *Ortolani test* is used to reduce a dislocated hip. This is performed by abducting and flexing the femur, and a palpable low-frequency clunk is noted as the femoral head slides back into the acetabulum.

### 13.36 Answers

**A** **True** – Risk of gestational diabetes increases with maternal age, especially >40 years.

**B** **True** – Risk of molar pregnancy is increased in very young/very old women.

**C** **True** – Risk of ectopic pregnancy increases with increasing maternal age – 1.4% aged 21 years, ~4% aged 35 tears and 6.9% aged 44 years.

**D** **False** – Risk of NTD is not affected by maternal age.

### 13.37 Answers

**A** **True** – Increased risk of spontaneous twin pregnancy (dizygotic) with increasing maternal age.

**B** **False.**

**C** **True** – Medical complications: women over 35 are twice as likely as women in their 20s to develop hypertension and diabetes in pregnancy, and are at increased risk of thromboembolic disease.

**D** **True.**

### 13.38 Answers

**A** **False** – See 13.36C.

**B** **False** – Risk of placenta previa increases with increasing maternal age – women in their 40s are eight times as likely as women in their 20s.

**C** **False** – See 13.37A.

**D** **True** – The risk of trophoblastic disease is increased in women over the age of 35 years.

Note:

• Fertility declines from the early 30s.

A **False** – Although the risk of placental abruption increases with maternal age, this is related to parity and is independent of maternal age.

B **True.**

C **False** – Increased risk of delivery before 37 completed weeks in women over the age of 35 years.

D **True** – Older women have increased risk of fetal distress in labour, prolonged second stage and delivery by caesarean section. Also, neonate has increased risk of admission to SCBU. Perinatal mortality is, however, not increased.

**M1.1** CA-125 levels are elevated in the following:

    A Ovarian teratomas.
    B Ovarian hyperstimulation syndrome.
    C Endometroid adenocarcinoma of the ovary.
    D Pelvic inflammatory disease.

**M1.2** Dermoid cysts:

    A Are mature ovarian teratomas.
    B Contain immature neural tissue.
    C Are the commonest ovarian tumours in childhood.
    D Are bilateral in 10–15% of women.

**M1.3** Granulosa cell tumours:

    A May present with isosexual precocious puberty.
    B May present with post-menopausal bleeding.
    C Are associated with endometrial hyperplasia and carcinoma.
    D Typically present with hirsutism and amenorrhoea.

**M1.4** The following are associated with an increased risk of developing endometrial cancer:

    A Diabetes mellitus.
    B Ovarian dysgerminoma.
    C Family history of breast or lung cancer.
    D Continuous combined HRT.

**M1.5** With respect to the BRCA1 and BRCA2 genes:

    A The risk of ovarian cancer associated with BRCA1 mutations is lower than that associated with BRCA2 mutations.
    B BRCA1 mutations are associated with an increased risk of lung cancer.
    C BRCA1 mutations are associated with an increased risk of colorectal and prostate cancer.
    D BRCA2 mutations are responsible for the majority of hereditary ovarian cancers.

**M1.6** The following are absolute contraindications to the use of the combined oral contraceptive pill:

A Prosthetic heart valves.
B Sickle cell disease.
C Active liver disease.
D Age under 14 years.

**M1.7** The following drugs reduce the efficacy of the combined oral contraceptive pill:

A Griseofulvin.
B Rifampicin.
C Warfarin.
D Indomethacin.

**M1.8** Bacterial vaginosis:

A Is characterized by a positive amine test.
B Is effectively treated with oral metronidazole.
C Is typically resistant to treatment with oral clindamycin.
D Is caused by *Trichomonas vaginalis*.

**M1.9** The following are recognized side effects of methyldopa therapy:

A Headache.
B Positive direct Coombs' test.
C Arrhythmias.
D Drowsiness.

**M1.10** Acute inversion of the uterus:

A Is a recognized complication of ergometrine administration.
B Causes tachycardia and hypertension.
C Can be treated by the O'Sullivan's hydrostatic pressure manoeuvre.
D May result from placenta acreta.

**M1.11** Umbilical cord prolapse is associated with:

A Induction of labour.
B Occipito-posterior position.
C Epidural anaesthesia.
D Preterm rupture of membranes.

**M1.12** Oligohydramnios is characteristically associated with:

A Twin-to-twin transfusion syndrome.
B Antenatal use of non-steroidal anti-inflammatory drugs.
C Fetal parvovirus infection.
D Neural tube defects.

**M1.13** There is a recognized association between intrauterine death of the fetus and:

A External cephalic version.
B Down syndrome.
C Gastroschisis.
D Bacterial vaginosis.

**M1.14** A 30-year-old woman is found to have a hydropic fetus at 25 weeks' gestation. The following are possible causes:

A Chromosomal anomaly.
B Alpha-thalassaemia.
C Sickle cell disease.
D Beta-thalassaemia major.

**M1.15** Tranexamic acid:

A Is contraindicated in women with thromboembolic disease.
B May result in a disturbance of colour vision.
C Causes constipation.
D Causes nausea and vomiting.

**M1.16** Gestrinone:

A Can virilize a female fetus.
B Is associated with a 2–3 kg weight gain.
C Is not associated with androgenic side effects.
D Suppresses ovulation.

**M1.17** Immune thrombocytopenia:

A Is frequently complicated by antepartum haemorrhage.
B Epidural analgesia is contraindicated if the platelet count is $>80 \times 10^9$/L.
C Caesarean section should be performed if platelet count is $<50\,000$/ml.
D Severity is assessed by quantifying antiplatelet antibodies.

**M1.18** The following drugs are absolutely contraindicated in breastfeeding:

A Heparin.
B Insulin.
C Warfarin.
D Carbimazole.

**M1.19** In pregnancy complicated by maternal insulin-dependent diabetes mellitus:

A There is an increased risk of sacral agenesis.
B There is an increased risk of IUGR.
C If glycaemic control is good, home delivery may be permitted.
D Fetal polycythaemia is more common.

**M1.20** The following are characteristic of the fetal hydantoin syndrome:

A Hypoplasia of distal phalanges and nails.
B Neural tube defects.
C Growth restriction.
D Learning disability.

**M1.21** Phaeochromocytoma complicating pregnancy:

A Is associated with glucose intolerance.
B Is associated with a ~50% fetal loss rate.
C Is associated with increased urinary excretion of vanillylmandelic acid.
D Is a recognized cause of pre-eclampsia.

**M1.22** Pemphigoid (Herpes) gestationis:

A Typically spares the umbilicus.
B Bullae do not occur.
C May be associated with poor fetal outcome.
D Neonatal disease does not occur.

**M1.23** The following drugs may exacerbate skeletal muscle weakness in a woman with myasthenia gravis:

A Lithium salts.
B Propranolol.
C Tetracycline.
D Oxytocin.

M1.24 A 30-year-old woman is known to have the antiphospholipid antibody syndrome:

A Her risk of miscarriage is reduced by treatment with aspirin.
B Heparin is ineffective in improving pregnancy outcome.
C Thrombocytopenia is a recognized complication.
D Thrombocytopenia is a recognized complication of heparin therapy.

M1.25 The following may cause acute pre-renal renal failure in pregnancy:

A Adrenocortical failure.
B Pyelonephritis.
C Broad ligament haematoma.
D Acute hydramnios.

M1.26 The following are recognized complications of massive blood transfusion:

A Hypocalcaemia.
B Hyperkalaemia.
C Thrombocytopenia.
D Haemoglobinuria.

M1.27 The following are recommended investigations in a woman who is otherwise fit and well with three successive first trimester miscarriages:

A Antiphospholipid antibody assays.
B Maternal and paternal karyotype.
C High vaginal and rectal swabs for culture.
D TORCH screen.

M1.28 There is a recognized association between Down syndrome and:

A Fifth finger clinodactily.
B Brachyceplaly.
C Exomphalos.
D Gastroschisis.

M1.29 Trisomy 18 is associated with:

A Choroid plexus cysts.
B Polyhydramnios.
C Oligohydramnios.
D Duodenal atresia.

**M1.30** Tetralogy of Fallot is characterized by:

    A Right ventricular outflow obstruction.
    B Left ventricular hypertrophy.
    C Cyanosis at birth.
    D Neonatal cyanosis during feeding or crying.

**M1.31** Turner's syndrome:

    A Is associated with impaired intellectual function.
    B The streak gonads should be excised at puberty to avert the risk of malignant change.
    C Is associated with fetal hydrops.
    D Is associated with cystic hygroma.

**M1.32** The following are recognized side effects of oxybutynin:

    A Blurred vision and dry mouth.
    B Drowsiness and diarrhea.
    C Palpitations and constipation.
    D Restlessness, disorientation and hallucinations.

**M1.33** With regards to the adverse effects of raloxifene:

    A Breast pain is associated with raloxifene treatment.
    B There is an increased risk of uterine fibroids.
    C The risk of endometrial hyperplasia is increased.
    D Thrombophlebitis is a recognized side effect.

**M1.34** Regarding antenatal and neonatal thyroid disease:

    A Hydrops fetalis may occur with maternal thyroxine intake.
    B Hydrops may occur with maternal Graves' disease.
    C Untreated neonatal hyperthyroidism leads to cretinism.
    D Pregnancy exacerbates Graves' disease.

**M1.35** In pregnant women with phenylketonuria:

    A A diet low in phenylalanine and tryptophan should be maintained.
    B Without treatment, there is an increased risk of fetal brain damage.
    C There is a 50% chance that the fetus is affected.
    D Chorionic villus sampling should be offered.

**M1.36** With respect to congenital adrenal hyperplasia:

    A ACTH levels are reduced.
    B Testosterone levels are elevated.
    C 17-alpha-hydroxyprogesterone levels are increased.
    D Aldosterone levels may be reduced, causing a salt losing syndrome.

**M1.37** Androgen insensitivity syndrome:

    A Plasma testosterone concentrations are within the normal range for males.
    B Plasma oestrogen is undetectable.
    C Testes are present and may be found in the abdomen, inguinal canal or labia.
    D There is an increased risk of malignancy in the testes and they should be removed after puberty.

**M1.38** The following are recognized long-term consequences of the polycystic ovary syndrome:

    A Increased risk of hypertension.
    B Increased risk of osteoporosis.
    C Increased risk of cervical cancer.
    D Increased risk of deep vein thrombosis.

**M1.39** The following are recognized side effects of clomiphene citrate:

    A Menorrhagia.
    B Amenorrhoea.
    C Abdominal discomfort.
    D Breast tenderness.

**M1.40** The following drugs can cause hirsutism:

    A Finasteride.
    B Gestrinone.
    C Cyproterone acetate.
    D Gestodene.

**M1.41** Anorexia nervosa:

    A Is associated with low TSH levels.
    B Amenorrhoea may occur before weight loss.
    C Is associated with low serum oestradiol levels.
    D The progesterone challenge test is typically positive.

**M1.42** The following are recognized side effects of bromocriptine therapy:

A Raynaud's phenomenon.
B Pleural effusion.
C Psychomotor disturbance.
D Headache.

**M1.43** In women who were exposed to diethylstilboestrol in utero:

A The risk of miscarriage is increased.
B Pregnancy rates are decreased.
C The risk of ectopic pregnancy is increased.
D The risk of preterm delivery is unchanged.

**M1.44** Toxoplasmosis in a pregnant woman:

A Causes fetal intracranial calcification.
B The risk of fetal infection falls with increasing gestational age.
C The risk of fetal damage falls with increasing gestational age.
D Is associated with chorioretinitis.

**M1.45** Fetal and neonatal cytomegalovirus infection:

A Is the commonest congenital infection in the UK.
B Can be diagnosed in the neonate by culture of urine.
C Does not occur if the mother is immune prior to pregnancy.
D 90% of fetuses are affected in primary maternal infections.

**M1.46** 3A 30-year-old woman is screened for syphilis at 14 weeks' gestation with the following results: VDRL – negative; FTA-ABS – positive:

A These results are consistent with treated syphilis.
B This may represent a biological false positive.
C There is no risk of congenital syphilis.
D The tests should be repeated 6 weeks later for confirmation.

**M1.47** A 30-year-old school teacher has come into contact with a 4-year-old with Fifth disease at 16 weeks' gestation. She presents 4 days after contact:

A The 4-year-old is highly infectious.
B If she is parvovirus B19 IgG positive, she should be reassured.
C If she is parvovirus B19 IgM and IgG negative, serology should be repeated in 1 week.
D If she subsequently becomes parvovirus B19 IgM positive, fetal blood sampling will be required to diagnose fetal infection.

**M1.48** An HIV-positive woman with her HIV-negative partner are planning a pregnancy:

A IVF is unethical if the couple are subfertile.
B Artificial insemination with washed sperm should be offered.
C The risk of vertical transmission in the absence of antiretroviral therapy is 5%.
D The couple should be offered artificial insemination around the time of ovulation.

**M1.49** With respect to the long-term risks and benefits of HRT:

A Use of HRT for 5 years from the age of 40 is associated with an increased risk of breast cancer.
B Use of HRT for 10 years from the age of 50 is associated with a significant reduction in the risk of hip fractures.
C Sequential combined HRT is associated with a reduction in endometrial cancer risk.
D Continuous combined HRT is associated with increased endometrial cancer risk.

**M1.50** With respect to HRT and breast cancer:

A Conjugated equine oestrogen is associated with a lower risk of breast cancer compared to oestradiol valerate.
B Continuous combined HRT is associated with a lower risk of breast cancer compared to sequential combined HRT.
C Use of medroxyprogesterone acetate is associated with lower risk of breast cancer when compared to norethisterone.
D Use of transdermal oestrogen is not associated with an increased risk of breast cancer.

M1.51 The tension-free vaginal tape:

A Is inserted at the level of the proximal urethra.
B At 1 year, has a similar success rate to the Burch colposuspension.
C Carries a 0.5% risk of bladder injury.
D Is typically inserted under local or regional anaesthesia.

M1.52 Duloxetine:

A Is a serotonin re-uptake inhibitor.
B Is an alpha-adrenergic antagonist.
C Results in increased activity in the urethral sphincter.
D Is effective treatment for detrusor instability.

M1.53 In a woman with choriocarcinoma, the following are associated with a worse prognosis:

A Age <25 years.
B Choriocarcinoma occurring after a normal pregnancy.
C Interval >12 months between antecedent pregnancy and chemotherapy.
D Blood group O or A.

M1.54 A 30-year-old woman is thought to have an ectopic pregnancy on transvaginal ultrasound scanning:

A At laparoscopy, salpingotomy should be performed if the other tube appears normal.
B Laparoscopic management is associated with a greater incidence of persistent trophoblastic tissue compared to laparotomy.
C Laparoscopic salpingotomy is associated with a significantly greater rate of repeat ectopic pregnancy compared to laparotomy and salpingotomy.
D The rate of subsequent intrauterine pregnancy does not differ significantly between laparoscopic procedures and laparotomy.

M1.55 In the diagnosis of endometriosis:

A The symptom complex of dysmenorrhoea, deep dyspareunia and infertility is diagnostic of endometriosis.
B MRI scan of the pelvis is a useful non-invasive investigation.
C CA-125 levels are typically >1000 U.
D A raised CA-125 identifies a subgroup of women who may benefit from early laparoscopy.

**M1.56** With regards to transection of the ureters recognized during laparotomy:

A End-to-end anastomosis is contraindicated.

B Repair should be performed using non-absorbable sutures.

C The Boari flap procedure is a recognized method of treatment.

D The site of injury should be drained and repair delayed for 2 weeks.

**M1.57** The following are recognized contraindications to the use of regional analgesia during labour:

A Maternal platelet count <150 000/ml.

B Active maternal haemorrhage.

C Untreated maternal febrile illness.

D Severe hypertension.

**M1.58** Hereditary non-polyposis colorectal cancer syndrome:

A Is inherited as an autosomal dominant trait.

B Is associated with an increased risk of endometrial cancer.

C Is associated with an increased risk of ovarian cancer.

D The majority of colorectal cancers occur in the rectum.

# Answers

**M1.1  Answers**

A  False.
B  True.
C  True.
D  True.

Note: Increased CA-125:

* Non-malignant causes: endometriosis, pelvic inflammatory disease, uterine fibroids, pregnancy, liver cirrhosis, tuberculous peritonitis, pelvic irradiation.
* Malignant causes: ovarian cancer, liver cancer, lung cancer, breast cancer, colon cancer, pancreatic cancer, endometrial cancer, cervical cancer.

**M1.2  Answers**

A  **True** – Mature cystic teratoma.
B  **False** – Immature neural tissue is an indication of malignancy.
C  **True.**
D  **True** – Bilateral in ~10% of cases.

**M1.3  Answers**

A  **True** – Present with isosexual precocious puberty, menorrhagia and irregular bleeding, post-menopausal bleeding secondary to oestrogens.
B  **True.**
C  **True** – Associated with endometrial hyperplasia and carcinoma, and with acute abdominal pain because of their tendency to rupture.
D  **False.**

**M1.4  Answers**

A  True.
B  False.
C  False.
D  False.

Note:

* Risk factors for endometrial cancer: obesity, nulliparity, late menopause/early menarche, PCOS, unopposed oestrogen therapy or endogenous oestrogen from granulosa cell tumour, tamoxifen therapy, diabetes mellitus, hypertension, personal or family history of breast or colon cancer.

**M1.5  Answers**

**A  False** – BRCA1 is responsible for 90% of hereditary ovarian cancers. Cumulative risk of developing ovarian cancer by age of 70 years is 30–60%. BRCA2 is responsible for 5–10% of hereditary ovarian cancers, with a cumulative risk of developing the disease by age of 70 years of 15–20%.

**B  False.**

**C  True.**

**D  False** – See A.

Note:

- BRCA1 is responsible for 50% of hereditary breast cancers. The cumulative risk of developing breast cancer by the age of 70 years is 80–90% in BRCA1 mutation carriers.
- BRCA2 is responsible for 40% of hereditary breast cancers. The cumulative risk of developing breast cancer by the age of 70 years is 80–90%.


**M1.6  Answers**

**A  False.**

**B  False.**

**C  True.**

**D  False.**

Note: Conditions for which COCP use is associated with unacceptable health risks (WHO Group 4):

- Previous thrombosis, ischemic heart disease.
- Cardiomyopathies, active Kawasaki disease.
- BMI >39, BP >160/100.
- Severe diabetes mellitus.
- Focal migraine.
- Thrombophilia.
- 4 weeks before major surgery to 2 weeks after full mobility.
- Active liver disease.
- Severe inflammatory bowel disease.
- Undiagnosed genital tract bleeding/pregnancy.
- Acute porphyria/SLE.
- Uncorrected valvular heart disease.
- TIAs/cerebral haemorrhage.
- Altitude >4500 m.
- Trophoblastic disease – until HCG undetectable.
- Hyperprolactinaemia (seek specialist advice).


**M1.7  Answers**

**A  True.**

**B  True** – For rifampicin/rifambutin use additional contraception for at least 4 weeks after stopping treatment.

**C  False.**

**D  False.**

Note:

- Drugs that reduce efficacy of COCP: carbamazepine, phenytoin (*not* valproate), griseofulvin, phenobarbital, primidone, rifampicin (and rifabutin), modafinil – take additional contraceptive precautions during use and for 7 days after use, starting next packet without a break if 7 days runs beyond the end of a packet.

## M1.8 Answers

**A** True.

**B** True.

**C** False – Sensitive to metronidazole/clindamycin. Topical/systemic therapy effective.

**D** False – There is an alteration in the vaginal microbial environment with a reduction in *Lactobaccilus* sp and an increase in facultative and anaerobic bacteria – *G. vaginalis/Bacteroides* sp/*Mobiluncus* sp.

Note:

- Bacterial vaginosis is associated with increased vaginal pH to 4.5–7.0.

## M1.9 Answers

**A** True.

**B** True.

**C** False.

**D** True.

Note: Side effects of methyldopa:

- CVS – bradycardia, exacerbation of angina, postural hypotension, oedema, myocarditis/pericarditis.
- CNS – sedation, headache, nightmares, depression/mild psychosis, parkinsonism, Bell's palsy.
- Blood – haemolytic anaemia (direct Coombs' test is positive), bone marrow suppression.

## M1.10 Answers

**A** False – Risk factors for acute inversion of the uterus include primiparity, fundal placenta, macrosomia and use of oxytocin. Recent data have not shown an association with placenta acreta.

**B** False – Presents with abdominal pain, PPH and/or shock in the presence of an inverted (vaginally) or indented (abdominally) uterus.

**C** True – Hydrostatic replacement (O'Sullivan's technique) involves manually sealing the introitus as sterile fluid is instilled into the vagina and is effective.

**D** False.

## M1.11 Answers

**A** True.

**B** False.

**C** False.

**D** True.

Note:

- Risk factors for umbilical cord prolapse: breech presentation, high head at onset of labour, multiple pregnancy, high parity, preterm labour, polyhydramnios, obstetric manipulations such as forceps delivery, artificial rupture of membranes.

## MI.12 Answers

- **A** **True** – More common in multiple pregnancy. In twin-to-twin transfusion syndrome, the donor twin typically has oligohydramnios.
- **B** **True** – NSAIDs reduce fetal urine output and are associated with oligohydramnios.
- **C** **False.**
- **D** **False.**

Note:

- Oligohydramnios causes: PPROM, IUGR, post-maturity, fetal anomalies (renal agenesis/
dysplasia, polycystic kidneys, urinary tract obstruction), chromosomal anomaly, fetal infection.

## MI.13 Answers

- **A** **True.**
- **B** **True.**
- **C** **True.**
- **D** **False.**

Note: Causes of intrauterine fetal death:

- Placental: IUGR, placental abruption, twin-to-twin transfusion syndrome, placental infarction, feto-maternal haemorrhage, trauma including ECV.
- Maternal systemic illness: diabetes mellitus, hypertensive disorders, maternal infections causing septicaemia and hypotension, thrombophilias such as SLE/antiphospholipid antibody syndrome.
- Fetal causes: malformations, chromosomal anomalies, viral and bacterial infections – parvovirus, TORCH, listeriosis, immune haemolytic disease, cord accidents, fetal metabolic disorders.

## MI.14 Answers

- **A** **True.**
- **B** **True.**
- **C** **False** – Fetus is not anaemic in sickle cell disease.
- **D** **False** – Fetus is not anaemic in chromosomal anoalies (trisomies/Turner's/triploidy).

Note:

- Causes of non-immune fetal hydrops: idiopathic (30%), infections (parvovirus B19, syphilis, CMV, toxoplasmosis, herpes simplex, leptospirosis, Chagas disease), anaemia (secondary to fetal infection, homozygous alpha-thalassaemia [not beta-thalassaemia], chronic feto-maternal haemorrhage, twin-to-twin transfusion).

## M1.15 Answers

**A True.**

**B True** – Side effects are nausea/vomiting/diarrhoea; disturbance in colour vision – discontinue therapy.

**C False.**

**D True** – See B.

Note:

- Not associated with an increased risk of DVT.

## M1.16 Answers

**A True** – Can virilize a female fetus, therefore barrier contraception is essential.

**B True** – Associated with 2–3 kg weight gain and GI disturbance.

**C False** – Gestrinone is associated with angrogenic side effects (milder than danazol).

**D True.**

## M1.17 Answers

**A False** – Spontaneous antepartum haemorrhage is uncommon.

**B False** – Regional anaesthesia is safe if counts are stable and >80 x 10⁹/L.

**C False** – C/S for obstetric reasons only and is unsafe at platelet count of 50 000/ml.

**D False** – Assay for antiplatelet antibodies not widely available and not useful in assessing disease severity.

Note:

- Treatment for immune thrombocytopenia is required if symptomatic (counts <20 x 10⁹/L).
- Corticosteroids are first-line treatment. Splenectomy should be avoided in pregnancy. I.v. gamma-globulin may be used in resistant cases.

## M1.18 Answers

**A False.**

**B False.**

**C False.**

**D False.**

Note:

- No drug is absolutely contraindicated – need to balance potential risks and benefits and the availability of alternative therapies.
- The only drugs known to carry a serious risk of harming the breastfed baby are antithyroid agents. The concentration of propylthiouracil may be higher in milk than in maternal plasma.

**M1.19 Answers**

    **A** **True** – 2–5x increase in risk of congenital anomalies, especially neural tube defects, cardiac anomalies (transposition of the great vessels), renal anomalies and sacral agenesis (caudal regression syndrome).

    **B** **True** – Increased risk of IUGR is associated with maternal hypertension + superimposed pre-eclampsia and nephropathy.

    **C** **False** – High risk labour/delivery – home delivery is *not* appropriate.

    **D** **True** – Polycythaemia is a recognized neonatal complication.

**M1.20 Answers**

    **A** True.

    **B** False.

    **C** True.

    **D** True.

Note:

- Major anomalies of fetal hydantoin syndrome include heart defects, cleft lip or palate, skeletal malformations and microcephaly, IUGR and learning disability.
- Minor malformations include strabismus, hypertelorism, distal digital hypoplasia, nail hypoplasia, clubfoot, broad nasal bridge and abnormal dermatoglyphic patterns.

**M1.21 Answers**

    **A** **True** – Presents in pregnancy with hypertensive crisis/paroxysmal hypertension ± cerebral haemorrhage or heart failure. May also present with circulatory collapse following delivery, palpitations, anxiety, headache, vomiting and glucose intolerance.

    **B** **True** – Fetal loss rate 15–50%.

    **C** **True** – Elevated urinary excretion of catecholamines and their metabolites such as vanillylmandelic acid is diagnostic. False-positive results may occur in women on methyldopa or labetalol.

    **D** **False** – Not a cause of pre-eclampsia.

**M1.22 Answers**

    **A** **False** – Pemphigoid (herpes) gestationis starts *within umbilicus* and spreads to involve limbs, palms and soles.

    **B** **False** – Presents with clusters of vesicles and bullae and is associated with other autoimmune diseases and HLA-B8 and DR3.

    **C** **True** – Possible increased risk of adverse perinatal outcome – monitor fetal growth and well-being.

    **D** **False** – 5% of neonates may develop bullous lesions.

## M1.23 Answers

**A** True.
**B** True.
**C** True.
**D** False.

Note:
*   Drugs that may cause or exacerbate muscle weakness in myasthenia gravis: magnesium salts, aminoglycosides, propranolol, tertracycline, barbiturates, lithium salts, penicillamine, quinine, procainamide, halothane, polymyxin B.

## M1.24 Answers

**A** **False** – A combination of aspirin and heparin significantly improves live birth rates in women with recurrent miscarriage and antiphospholipid syndrome. Treatment with aspirin alone does not seem to improve live birth rates but there remains some controversy.
**B** **False.**
**C** **True** – Thrombocytopenia is a recognized complication of antiphospholipid antibody syndrome.
**D** **True** – Thrombocytopenia is also a complication of treatment with heparin.

## M1.25 Answers

**A** **True** – Adrenocortical failure is usually secondary to inadequate steroid cover in women on long-term corticosteroid therapy.
**B** **True** – Septic shock is secondary to pyelonephritis.
**C** **False** – Acute hydramnios and broad ligament haematoma cause *post*-renal renal failure by ureteric obstruction.
**D** **False.**

## M1.26 Answers

**A** **True.**
**B** **True** – Hyperkalaemia from high potassium in stored cells.
**C** **True** – Thrombocytopenia and coagulopathy due to depleted clotting factors.
**D** **False** – Haemoglobinuria does not occur.

## M1.27 Answers

**A** **True** – Screening for antiphospholipid antibodies on two occasions at least 6 weeks apart.
**B** **True** – Karyotype of couple.
**C** **False** – Genital tract swabs and TORCH screen not recommended.
**D** **False.**

## M1.28 Answers

**A** True.
**B** True.
**C** True.
**D** False.

Note:

- 55% of neonates with Down syndrome have structural anomaly.
- Cardiac anomalies – atrioventricular canal defects.
- GI anomalies – duodenal atresia, exomphalos, Hirschprung's disease.
- Urinary tract/limb defects (fifth finger clinodactily)/congenital cataract.
- Brachycephaly/upslanting palpebral fissures/Brushfield spots/epicanthic folds/open mouth with protruding tongue.

## M1.29 Answers

**A** True.
**B** True.
**C** True.
**D** False.

Note:

- Trisomy 18 is associated with multiple anomalies, including: early onset IUGR, rockerbottom feet, clenched fist, overlapping fingers, choroid plexus cyst, two vessel cord, increased nuchal translucency, oligohydramnios, polyhydramnios, renal/cardiac/CNS/skeletal anomalies.

## M1.30 Answers

**A** **True** – Tetralogy of Fallot is characterized by ventricular septal defect, right ventricular outflow obstruction (pulmonary infundibular stenosis), overriding aorta, right ventricular hypertrophy.
**B** **False.**
**C** **False** – Neonate is pink at birth.
**D** **True** – Neonate becomes cyanosed with crying or feeding – cyanosis develops and progresses over the first few weeks of life.

Note:

- Cyanosis occurs at rest in childhood with 'squatting' behaviour – traps venous blood in legs, increases resistance in aorta, hence reducing right-to-left shunt.
- 95% survival after corrective surgery.

## M1.31 Answers

**A** **False** – 45,X0. Normal intellectual development.
**B** **False** – Streak ovaries with primary amenorrhoea (ovarian dysgenesis) but no increase in risk of ovarian malignancy.
**C** **True** – Turner's syndrome is associated with increased nuchal translucency, coarctation of the aorta, atrial septal defects, cystic hygroma, fetal hydrops.
**D** **True.**

### M1.32 Answers

**A** True.
**B** True.
**C** True.
**D** True.

Note:
- Side effects of oxybutynin include: nausea, constipation, diarrhoea and abdominal discomfort; dry mouth (88%); blurred vision; voiding difficulties and urinary retention; headache, dizziness, drowsiness, restlessness and disorientation; rash, dry skin, photosensitivity; arrhythmia, angioedema.

### M1.33 Answers

**A** False – Raloxifene is a SERM and has antioestrogen effects on the genital tract and breast. Therefore, it is not associated with breast pain, PMB or endometrial hyperplasia.
**B** False.
**C** False – See A.
**D** True – Causes leg cramps, thrombophlebitis, hot flushes, peripheral oedema and flu-like symptoms. Also associated with GI disturbance, headache and hypertension.

### M1.34 Answers

**A** False – Thyroxine does not cross the placenta in significant quantities and does not cause fetal toxicity.
**B** True – Maternal thyroid-stimulating antibodies in Graves' disease cross the placenta and can cause fetal thyrotoxicosis with heart failure and hydrops.
**C** False – *Hypo*thyroidism causes cretinism.
**D** False – Autoimmune diseases typically get better during pregnancy.

### M1.35 Answers

**A** True – Women with PKU need to have disease adequately controlled before conception.
**B** True – Risk of fetal brain damage by transplacental passage of phenylpyruvate products.
**C** False – Autosomal recessive, deficiency of phenylalanine hydroxylase. If partner is a carrier, 1:4 chance of affected fetus.
**D** False – Not an indication for CVS.

Note:
- Treat infant with PKU with low phenylalanine/tryptophan diet within 20 days of birth and then life-long or at least into adulthood. Good outcome.

## M1.36 Answers

A **False** – Raised ACTH, 17-alpha-hydroxyprogesterone, progesterone, androstendione, testosterone in congenital adrenal hyperplasia.

B **True.**

C **True.**

D **True** – Salt losing syndrome may present with vomiting and failure to thrive secondary to aldosterone deficiency.

Note:

- Commonest enzyme defect is 21-hydroxylase deficiency (90% of cases), resulting in a failure of conversion of 17-alpha-hydroxyprogesterone to 11-deoxycortisol; 17-hydroxyprogesterone and progesterone levels are increased with subsequent conversion to androstendione and testosterone with resulting masculinization of the female fetus.

## M1.37 Answers

A **True.**

B **False** – Oestrogen levels overlap between male and female range.

C **True.**

D **True** – Increased risk of cancer in testes – gonadectomy recommended after puberty + oestrogen replacement therapy.

## M1.38 Answers

A **True.**

B **False.**

C **False.**

D **False.**

Note: Long-term sequelae of PCOS:

- Increased risk of hypertension.
- Cardiovascular disease – mortality is not significantly increased although women with PCOS have abnormal lipid profiles.
- Increased risk of endometrial cancer (five-fold) but not cervical cancer.
- Risk of VTE not increased.

## M1.39 Answers

A **True.**

B **False.**

C **True.**

D **True.**

Note: Side effects of clomiphene:

- Visual disturbance – withdraw.
- OHSS.
- Hot flushes, headache, depression, insomnia, convulsions and dizziness.
- Breast tenderness, intermenstrual bleeding, menorrhagia.
- Nausea, vomiting, abdominal discomfort.
- Hair loss.

## M1.40 Answers

**A** False.
**B** True.
**C** False.
**D** False.

Note:

- Exogenous/iatrogenic androgens cause hirsutism: testosterone, anabolic steroids, androgenic progestogens, danazol.
- Phenytoin, cortisone, minoxidil, diazoxide and cyclosporin A alter the texture and extent of hair growth – the pattern is non-androgenic and is referred to as hypertrichosis.

## M1.41 Answers

**A** False – TSH and T4 levels are normal but T3 and reverse T3 are elevated.
**B** True – Amenorrhoea frequently pre-dates weight loss.
**C** True – Oestradiol and progesterone levels are low.
**D** False – Progesterone challenge test is typically negative.

## M1.42 Answers

**A** True.
**B** True.
**C** True.
**D** True.

Note:

- Side effects of bromocriptine: nausea; vomiting; headache; postural hypotension; constipation; dizziness; drowsiness; Raynaud's phenomenon; psychiatric symptoms; especially aggression; pleural effusion; retroperitomeal fibrosis reported.

## M1.43 Answers

**A** True – Risk of spontaneous miscarriage is doubled.
**B** False – Fecundity (pregnancy rates) is not affected.
**C** True – Risk of ectopic pregnancy is increased up to 10-fold.
**D** False – Risk of preterm labour is increased.

## M1.44 Answers

**A** True.
**B** False – Risk of fetal infection increases while risk of affection decreases with increasing gestational age.
**C** True.
**D** True.

Note: Fetal risks associated with toxoplasmosis:

- Microcephaly, hydrocephalus, intracranial calcification.
- Spontaneous first trimester miscarriage, chorioretinitis, IUGR.

## M1.45 Answers

**A** **True** – CMV is the commonest congenital viral infection in pregnancy.
**B** **True** – Excreted in urine.
**C** **False** – Fetal infection occurs with primary as well as re-activated infection.
**D** **False** – 5–10% of infected neonates are symptomatic at birth. Of asymptomatic neonates, 5–15% develop symptoms by the second year of life, usually sensorineural deafness.

## M1.46 Answers

**A** **True** – VDRL/RPR (rapid plasma reagin) – cardiolipin antibody tests. Positive in untreated secondary/latent/tertiary syphilis, become negative with treatment. Treponemal antibody tests – TPHA (*Treponema pallidum* haemagglutination) and FTA-ABS (fluorescent treponemal antibody – absorption test) remain positive even with adequate treatment.
**B** **False.**
**C** **False** – FTA-ABS becomes positive before VDRL or RPR. The woman may therefore still be infected with the risk of congenital infection.
**D** **False** – No indication for repeating test.

## M1.47 Answers

**A** **False** – Rash does not occur until 17–18 days after infection and about 5 days after the disappearance of virus from serum and respiratory droplets. Patients presenting with the clinical infection are usually no longer infectious.
**B** **True** – IgG detectable by the seventh day of illness and persists for life. Conveys lasting immunity to infection. Therefore reassure.
**C** **False** – IgM is detectable 3 days after the onset of symptoms and may persist for up to 6 months. If IgM negative at the first test, it should be repeated 2–3 weeks later depending on timing of exposure.
**D** **False** – If maternal infection confirmed, serial ultrasound scans for the early detection of hydrops – follow-up scans for up to 12 weeks after confirmed maternal infection.

## M1.48 Answers

**A** **False** – IVF treatment is ethically acceptable in subfertile couples given low vertical transmission rate (<2%) and life expectancy of parents taking HAART.
**B** **False** – As the partner is negative there is no need for sperm preparation.
**C** **False** – In the absence of treatment, risk of vertical transmission ~20%.
**D** **True** – Insemination around the time of ovulation is appropriate treatment.

## M1.49 Answers

A **False** – HRT in women with a premature menopause is not associated with an increased risk of breast cancer. Duration of oestrogen exposure appears to be the risk factor.

B **False** – Use of HRT for 5–10 years around the menopause does not confer enough protection to reduce the risk of hip fractures at the age of 79. HRT has to be taken life-long to be effective.

C **False** – Sequential combined HRT but *not* continuous combined HRT is associated with an increased risk of endometrial cancer.

D **False.**

## M1.50 Answers

A **False.**
B **False.**
C **False.**
D **False.**

Note:

- Risk of breast cancer does not differ significantly between specific oestrogens and progestagens, their doses or between continuous and sequential regimens.

## M1.51 Answers

A **False** – Uses a knitted prolene mesh tape placed at the mid-urethra.

B **True** – Similar success rates to colposuspension in RCTs. Complete dryness in 38% (TVT) and 40% (colposuspension) at 6 months.

C **False** – Carries an 8% risk of bladder injury.

D **True.**

## M1.52 Answers

A **True** – Duloxetine is a combined serotonin and noradrenaline re-uptake inhibitor.

B **False.**

C **True** – Increased synaptic concentrations of noradrenaline and 5-HT within the pudendal nerve results in increased stimulation of the urethral sphincter.

D **False** – Increases sphincter activity in the storage phase of the micturiction cycle and therefore used in the treatment of stress incontinence.

**M1.53 Answers**

    **A** **False** – Prognosis worse if aged >39 years or >para 4.

    **B** **True** – Prognosis worse after full-term pregnancy/spontaneous miscarriage; better after known molar pregnancy.

    **C** **True** – Better prognosis if interval between pregnancy and chemotherapy < 4 months, worse if >12 months.

    **D** **False** – Prognosis better in blood groups O and A, worse in blood groups B and AB.

**M1.54 Answers**

    **A** **False** – If other tube is normal, salpingectomy should be performed.

    **B** True – Higher rate of persistent trophoblastic tissue (12.2% vs 1.7%) if salpingotomy performed.

    **C** **False** – A trend towards a lower repeat ectopic pregnancy rate with laparoscopic salpingotomy.

    **D** **True** – No significant difference in subsequent intrauterine pregnancy rates compared to laparotomy.

Note:

* Laparoscopy is associated with: lower blood loss, lower analgesic requirement, shorter hospital stay, quicker post-op recovery, lower cost.

**M1.55 Answers**

    **A** **False** – Clinical diagnosis is unreliable as symptoms such as dysmenorrhoea and pelvic pain are common and there is a considerable overlap with conditions such as irritable bowel syndrome and PID.

    **B** **True** – MRI may be a useful non-invasive tool in the diagnosis of deep infiltrating endometriosis.

    **C** **False** – Serum CA-125 is *mildly* elevated in endometriosis but is of limited value as a screening or diagnostic test.

    **D** **True** – Raised CA-125 may identify a subgroup of women in whom early laparoscopy is warranted.

**M1.56 Answers**

    **A** **False** – For ureteric transection at the pelvic brim or above, end-to-end anastomosis should be performed over a Sialastic stent.

    **B** **False** – Repair should be performed by a trained urologist using fine absorpable interrupted sutures.

    **C** **True** – Damage at or below the level of the ureteric tunnel is best managed by re-implantation into the bladder. Injury higher up the pelvic side-wall is best managed by mobilizing the bladder to allow ureteric re-implantation without tension using a psoas hitch or Boari flap (a flap of bladder is elevated into which the ureter is re-implanted. The flap is then closed as a tube).

    **D** **False.**

**M1.57 Answers**

A **False** – Epidural contraindicated in maternal coagulopathy (inherited or acquired) but may be administered if platelet count >80 000/ml.

B **True.**

C **True** – Epidural contraindicated in maternal septicemia or untreated febrile illness.

D **False.**

Note:

- Other contraindications to epidural analgesia include patient refusal and infection at or near needle insertion site.

**M1.58 Answers**

A **True.**

B **True** – Autosomal dominant pre-disposition to colorectal cancer in addition to endometrial, ovarian, stomach, pancreatic, renal tract and small bowel cancers. 30–39% cumulative risk of developing endometrial cancer by the age of 70 years in HNPCC compared to ~3% in the general population, and these cancers occur 15 years earlier than the population peak of 65 years. The cumulative life-time risk of ovarian cancer in Lynch II syndrome is ~9% and is ~75% for colorectal cancer.

C **True.**

D **False** – 70% of tumours are proximal to the splenic flexure.

# Mock examination 2: Questions

**M2.1** With respect to staging of endometrial cancer:

    A Stage Ib – invasion of <50% of the myometrium.
    B Stage IIa – cervical stromal involvement.
    C Stage IIb – cervical glandular involvement.
    D Stage IIIb – vaginal metastases.

**M2.2** The progesterone-only oral contraceptive pill:

    A Is taken for 21 days with a 7-day break each month.
    B Suppresses ovulation in ~40% of cycles.
    C Efficacy is increased in over-weight women.
    D Efficacy increases with increasing age of user.

**M2.3** The following are recognized side effects of nifedipine therapy:

    A Hypertension.
    B Raynaud's phenomenon.
    C Palpitations.
    D Constipation.

**M2.4** Congenital abnormalities of the uterus are associated with:

    A Pre-eclampsia.
    B Polyhydramnios.
    C Renal tract anomalies.
    D Unstable lie of the fetus.

**M2.5** Continuous electronic fetal monitoring in labour:

    A Is associated with a lower rate of neonatal seizures.
    B Results in a significant reduction in the number of babies with low Apgar scores a 1 min.
    C Should be recommended if regional analgesia is used.
    D Should be recommended in all prolonged pregnancies (>42 complete weeks).

**M2.6** The following investigations are relevant in the investigation of the hydropic fetus:

A Paternal blood group.
B Maternal and paternal karyotype for balanced translocation.
C Fetal karyotype.
D PCR for fetal parvovirus infection.

**M2.7** Danazol:

A Is associated with musculoskeletal pains and breast tenderness.
B May cause hirsutism.
C Should not be administered for longer than 6 months.
D Is an androgenic antioestrogen and antiprogestogen.

**M2.8** Amniotic fluid embolism:

A Can be treated with heparin.
B Causes disseminated intravascular coagulation.
C Always results in fetal death.
D Presents with pleuritic chest pain and haemoptysis 24 hours after delivery.

**M2.9** The following are characteristic features of the fetal warfarin syndrome:

A Growth restriction.
B Gastroschisis.
C Stippled epiphyses.
D Neural tube defects.

**M2.10** The following cardiac conditions are associated with a high risk of maternal mortality:

A Pulmonary hypertension.
B Aortic stenosis.
C Mitral stenosis with atrial fibrillation.
D Hypertrophic obstructive cardiomyopathy.

**M2.11** The following are recognized features of septic miscarriage:

A Crepitus.
B Raised CRP.
C Hypothermia.
D Pyrexia.

**M2.12** There is a recognized association between Down syndrome and:

A Duodenal atresia.
B Hirschprung's.
C Advanced paternal age.
D Raised maternal serum AFP.

**M2.13** Maternal serum AFP levels are raised in:

A Antepartum haemorrhage.
B After amniocentesis.
C Women taking the combined oral contraceptive in early pregnancy.
D Choriocarcinoma.

**M2.14** A child with Klinefelter's syndrome:

A Is at increased risk of osteoporosis in the long term if untreated.
B Testosterone treatment can improve fertility.
C Has an impaired sense of smell.
D Is likely to be of short stature.

**M2.15** Turner's syndrome:

A Is associated with increased nuchal transluscency.
B Is associated with an increased risk of hypertension in adulthood.
C Is associated with an increased risk of Hashimoto.
D Nail hyperplasia is a characteristic feature.

**M2.16** Isolated renal pelvi-calyceal dilatation:

A Postnatal renal ultrasound should be performed within 24 hours in female infants.
B Is associated with vesicoureteric reflux.
C Postnatal renal ultrasound should be performed within 24 hours in a male infant with an enlarged bladder.
D Is associated with posterior urethral valves.

**M2.17** The following are recognized clinical manifestations of the polycystic ovary syndrome:

A Clitoral enlargement.
B Oligomenorrhoea.
C Secondary infertility.
D Primary infertility.

**M2.18** The following drugs are associated with hypertrichosis:

A Phenytoin.
B Diazoxide.
C Minoxidil.
D Finasteride.

**M2.19** The following endocrine disorders are associated with hyper-prolactinaemia:

A Cushing's disease.
B Cushing's syndrome.
C Acromegaly.
D Primary hypothyroidism.

**M2.20** In patients with anorexia nervosa:

A LH and FSH levels are elevated.
B Pituitary response to GnRH is suboptimal.
C There is loss of pulsatile release of GnRH.
D Serum prolactin is markedly elevated.

**M2.21** The following are recognized causes of secondary amenorrhoea:

A Cushing's syndrome.
B Hypothyroidism.
C Congenital adrenal hyperplasia.
D Kallman's syndrome.

**M2.22** With respect to the FIGO staging of ovarian cancer:

A Stage Ia – cancer restricted to both ovaries with negative peritoneal cytology.
B Stage IIIb – intrahepatic metastases.
C Stage IV – malignant pleural effusion.
D Stage IIa –metastases confined to the uterus and tubes only.

**M2.23** With respect to the side effects of chemotherapeutic agents for ovarian cancer:

A Carboplatin is more nephrotoxic than cisplatin.
B Forced diuresis reduces the incidence of nephrotoxicity in women receiving platinum agents.
C Ondansetron has been shown to significantly reduce the incidence of vomiting in women receiving platinum agents.
D Dexamethasone is useful in reducing chemotherapy-associated vomiting.

M2.24 In a 45-year-old woman with stage I endometrial cancer on endometrial sampling and MRI imaging:

A Total abdominal hysterectomy with ovarian conservation is acceptable management.

B Excision of vaginal cuff significantly reduces the risk of a vault recurrence.

C Postoperative oestrogen replacement is associated with increased risk of recurrence.

D Tubal ligation should be performed prior to hysterectomy to reduce the risk of intraoperative spill of tumour.

M2.25 Malignant melanoma of the vulva:

A Diameter of the tumour is the most important prognostic factor.

B Depth of invasion is the most important prognostic factor.

C Carries a better prognosis compared to other cutaneous melanomas.

D Chemotherapy is recommended treatment.

M2.26 Sarcoma botryoides:

A ~90% occur in children below the age of 5 years.

B Combination chemotherapy is recommended treatment.

C Are associated with in utero exposure to diethylstilboestrol.

D Typically present with a vaginal mass of grape-like vesicles.

M2.27 The low dose (20–35 µg ethinyloestradiol) combined oral contraceptive pill:

A Has a failure rate of 1/100 woman-years.

B Is associated with a significant increase in the risk of breast cancer in current users compared to never users.

C Should be discontinued at the age of 40 years in smokers.

D Provides adequate contraception to epileptics taking valproate.

M2.28 A woman who conceived with an intrauterine device in situ:

A The device should be removed as soon as possible to reduce the risk of miscarriage.

B The risk of congenital malformation is increased.

C The risk of preterm labour is increased.

D The risk of third-stage complications is increased.

M2.29 The administration of 600 mg mifepristone to a woman who is 8 weeks' pregnant:

A Results in a rise in plasma ACTH levels.
B Results in a fall in plasma cortisol levels.
C Results in a withdrawal of progesterone support to the decidua.
D Results in increased prostaglandin concentrations in the myometrium.

M2.30 In the management of a woman who has suffered an eclamptic fit:

A Treatment with magnesium sulphate is associated with a lower risk of recurrent seizures compared to treatment with diazepam.
B A loading dose of 4 g of magnesium sulphate should be administered over 2 minutes.
C In the event of further seizures, a further bolus dose of 4 g magnesium sulphate should be administered.
D The therapeutic range for magnesium sulphate is 2–4 mM.

M2.31 The following statements about breech delivery are true:

A Planned caesarean section has been shown in a randomized trial to be associated with a two-fold increase in maternal morbidity compared to planned vaginal delivery.
B Planned caesarean section is associated with lower perinatal morbidity compared to planned vaginal delivery.
C Lovset's manoeuvre is used to deliver the head.
D Wrigley's forceps are best suited for delivery of the after-coming head.

M2.32 A 30-year-old primigravida who has been the victim of infibulation is referred to the antenatal clinic at 14 weeks' gestation.

A A defibulation operation can be performed at 20 weeks' gestation.
B If the woman wishes, re-infibulation should be performed following delivery.
C The risk of puerperal sepsis is increased.
D A posterior midline episiotomy should be performed in the second stage.

M2.33 The following are indications for fetal echocardiography:

A History of congenital heart disease in the mother.
B Increased nuchal translucency thickness at 13 weeks' gestation.
C Raised maternal serum alpha-fetoprotein.
D Antenatal lithium therapy.

M2.34 With regards to preterm labour:

A In women with a previous history of bacterial vaginosis and preterm labour, treatment with metronidazole improves outcome.
B Bacterial enzymes such as collagenases may weaken the membranes, resulting in rupture and subsequent labour.
C Tocolysis is less likely to be successful in the presence of positive amniotic fluid microbiology.
D Rapid transplacental passage makes erythromycin the ideal antibiotic prophylaxis for preterm rupture of membranes.

M2.35 The use of intravenous ritodrine on its own is associated with:

A Hypokalaemia.
B Hypoglycaemia.
C Maternal tachycardia.
D Fetal tachycardia.

M2.36 The following are relative contraindications to endometrial resection:

A A 12-week size fibroid uterus.
B Failed response to the levonorgestrel-releasing intrauterine system.
C Woman desires amenorrhoea.
D Dysmenorrhoea.

M2.37 With respect to the medical management of endometriosis:

A A 6-month course of GnRH agonist is associated with a 6% loss of bone mineral density.
B Bone loss after a 6-month course of GnRH agonist is restored within 6 months of cessation of therapy.
C GnRH agonists are more effective than danazol.
D GnRH agonists are effective when administered by the oral route.

M2.38  DVT in pregnancy:

A  Is commoner in the right leg.
B  Is commoner in nulliparous women.
C  Is commoner in blood group O.
D  Should only be treated if it extends above the knee.

M2.39  The following conditions are typically exacerbated in pregnancy:

A  Rheumatoid arthritis.
B  Sarcoidosis.
C  Asthma.
D  Eczema.

M2.40  Liver disease in pregnancy:

A  Acute fatty liver of pregnancy typically presents in the first trimester.
B  Acute fatty liver of pregnancy is commoner in primigravidae.
C  Acute fatty liver of pregnancy is associated with hyperglycaemia.
D  Cholestasis of pregnancy is associated with fetal distress.

M2.41  In pregnancy complicated by maternal IDDM:

A  Maternal serum AFP concentrations are higher than in non-diabetics.
B  Maternal serum HCG concentrations are lower than in non-diabetics.
C  Maternal serum unconjugated oestriol concentrations are lower than in non-diabetics.
D  Preterm delivery is more common.

M2.42  Anaemia in sickle cell disease:

A  Responds well to folic acid.
B  Is usually megaloblastic.
C  Is associated with a normal MCV.
D  Can be treated with exchange transfusion.

**M2.43** With respect to thyroid function and thyroid disease in pregnancy:

    A Pregnancy is associated with a fall in thyroxine binding globulin concentrations.

    B The concentration of total T3 and T4 is unchanged in normal pregnancy.

    C The concentration of free T3 and T4 is unchanged in normal pregnancy.

    D Hyperthyroidism is associated with elevated TSH levels.

**M2.44** In early pregnancy:

    A A gestation sac can be identified by transabdominal scan when HCG >6000 IU/L.

    B A pseudo-sac is visualized in over 80% of ectopic pregnancies.

    C In a normal pregnancy, fetal heart should always demonstrable if CRL >6 mm.

    D In a normal pregnancy, fetal heart should always be detectable if sac diameter >30 mm.

**M2.45** With respect to molar pregnancy:

    A The lowest incidence is in women aged over 35 years.

    B There is a recognized geographical variation in incidence.

    C The recurrence risk is ~1:500.

    D The risk of choriocarcinoma is higher with complete moles compared to partial moles.

**M2.46** A 30-year-old woman is found to have a tubal ectopic pregnancy. The following features make her suitable for medical treatment:

    A Serum HCG level >10 000 IU/ml.

    B Demonstration of a fetal heart echo on transvaginal scan.

    C Diameter of ectopic pregnancy <2 cm.

    D Pulse of 110 bpm.

**M2.47** Listerosis:

    A Fetal disease is caused by transplacental transfer of antibodies.

    B May present with flu-like illness.

    C Is associated with meconium-stained liquor.

    D Late-onset neonatal disease presents with disseminated granulomas and septic shock.

M2.48  2A 24-year-old woman is found to have asymptomatic Group B streptococcal bacteriuria at 20 weeks' gestation:

A  Treatment should be deferred until the onset of labour.
B  Erythromycin is the treatment of choice.
C  A high vaginal swab should be performed for culture.
D  She is at increased risk of preterm delivery.

M2.49  An HIV-positive woman has just had a vaginal delivery following antenatal HAART:

A  The neonate should receive antiretroviral therapy for the first 4–6 weeks of life.
B  An HIV antibody test should be performed on the child at 3 and 6 weeks.
C  The neonate should be screened for HIV infection at birth using PCR.
D  An HIV antibody test should be performed on the child at 18 months of age if earlier screening is negative.

M2.50  With respect to the innervation of the urinary bladder and the control of micturiction:

A  The detrusor is innervated mainly by sympathetic fibres from the S2,3,4 spinal segments.
B  The extrinsic urethral sphincter mechanism is under voluntary control.
C  Micturiction is inhibited by higher cortical centres.
D  The parasympathetic nerves supplying the bladder form synapses within the detrusor muscle.

M2.51  The following are consistent with a diagnosis of interstitial cystitis:

A  Reduced bladder capacity.
B  Culture of coliforms on MSU.
C  Ulceration of the bladder mucosa at cystoscopy.
D  Presence of involuntary detrusor contractions on cystometry.

M2.52  The use of raloxifene in post-menopausal women has been shown to be associated with the following effects:

A  Increased bone mineral density.
B  A significant reduction in the risk of vertebral fractures.
C  A significant reduction in the risk of breast cancer.
D  A significant reduction in the risk of endometrial cancer.

M2.53  Tamoxifen:

A  May re-activate endometriosis in post-menopausal women.
B  Is associated with a 10% reduction in breast cancer recurrence.
C  As adjuvant treatment, is associated with a 10% reduction in breast cancer mortality.
D  Is associated with an increased risk of deep venous thrombosis.

M2.54  With respect to lasers:

A  Maximum permitted exposure limits must be observed.
B  The $CO_2$ laser is most appropriate for hysteroscopic surgery.
C  The Nd:YAG laser has a greater depth of penetration compared to the $CO_2$ laser.
D  The argon laser produces visible light.

M2.55  A 47-year-old woman is undergoing laparotomy for ovarian cancer.

A  Subcutaneous heparin 5000 U twice daily is superior to 'no treatment' in preventing venous thromboembolism.
B  Subcutaneous heparin 5000 U three times daily carries a greater risk of haemorrhage than 5000 U twice daily.
C  Oral warfarin is easier to reverse than subcutaneous heparin.
D  Calf compression has been shown to significantly reduce the risk of venous thromboembolism.

M2.56  The following are remnants of the Wolffian (mesonephric) duct:

A  Epoophron.
B  Paroophron.
C  Hydatid of Morgani.
D  Gartner's duct.

M2.57  Haematocolpos:

A  Is typically associated with secondary amenorrhoea.
B  Presents with cyclical lower abdominal pain.
C  May present with acute urinary retention.
D  Is typically associated with uterus didelphys.

**M2.58** In a neonate with ambiguous genitalia:

A A thorough inspection of the external genitalia should be undertaken to determine sex.

B Karyotype is mandatory.

C Electrolytes should be measured to exclude a salt-losing syndrome.

D Turner's syndrome is a possible diagnosis.

# Answers

## M2.1 Answers

**A** **True** – Ib – <50% myometrial invasion.
**B** **False** – IIa – endocervical glandular involvement.
**C** **False** – IIb – endocervical stromal involvement.
**D** **True** – IIIb – vaginal metastases.

## M2.2 Answers

**A** **False** – One tablet daily taken from day 1 of the cycle and taken continuously. Should be taken at the same time every day and within 3 h at the most.
**B** **True** – Suppresses ovulation in ~40% of cycles; this is unpredictable and varies between cycles resulting in irregular menstruation.
**C** **False** – Efficacy may be reduced if increased weight >70 kg – consider double dose.
**D** **True**.

## M2.3 Answers

**A** False.
**B** False.
**C** True.
**D** True.

Note: Side effects of nifedipine:
- GI: nausea, constipation/diarrhoea, gum hyperplasia.
- GU: frequency of micturiction, impotence, gynaecomastia.
- CVS: tachycardia, palpitations, dizziness, oedema.
- CNS: eye pain, visual disturbance, headache, paraesthesia, tremor.

## M2.4 Answers

**A** False.
**B** False.
**C** True.
**D** True.

Note: Uterine anomalies associated with:
- Preterm delivery and malpresentation, including breech presentation and unstable lie.
- Increased risk of PPH.
- Increased risk of urinary tract anomalies.

## M2.5 Answers

**A** **True** – Associated with a significant reduction in neonatal seizures.
**B** **False** – No significant reduction in low Apgar scores at 1 min.
**C** **True.**
**D** **True.**

Note:

- Because of the risk of fetal acidosis, electronic fetal monitoring is recommended in high-risk labours (including those in which oxytocin is used, prolonged pregnancies, use of regional analgesia).

## M2.6 Answers

**A** **False.**
**B** **False.**
**C** **True.**
**D** **True.**

Note: Investigations in fetal hydrops:

- Maternal: FBC, U&E, LFT, urate, blood group + antibodies, Hb electrophoresis (depending on ethnic group), MSAFP, infection screen – TORCH + parvovirus B19 + syphilis + coxsackie, Kleihauer, GTT, lupus anticoagulant + anti-Ro antibodies if bradyarrhythmia.
- Fetal: detailed ultrasound scan, biophysical assessment, fetal blood sampling – FBC group, Coomb's test, karyotype, Hb electrophoresis if required + PCR-based infection screen/antibody screen for infection.

## M2.7 Answers

**A** **False.**
**B** **True** – Associated with androgenic side effects: weight gain of 2–4 kg with 3-months' treatment, acne, hirsutism, seborrhoea, irritability, musculoskeletal pains, fatigue, hot flushes and breast atrophy.
**C** **True** – The recommended duration of treatment is up to 6 months.
**D** **True** – Synthetic androgen with antioestrogenic and antiprogestogenic activity.

## M2.8 Answers

**A** **True** – If diagnosed before death, management is supportive – give $O_2$, maintain circulation, treat DIC and manage in ITU. Discuss heparin therapy with haematologist.
**B** **True.**
**C** **False** – Fetal survival 79% with 39% of these neurologically intact.
**D** **False** – Criteria for diagnosis include acute hypotension or cardiac arrest, acute hypoxia, coagulopathy, onset during labour, C/S or within 30 minutes of delivery and absence of other.

## M2.9 Answers

**A** True.
**B** False.
**C** True.
**D** False.

Note:
- Warfarin embryopathy occurs in 15–25% of pregnancies when used in the first trimester.
- Most common features are nasal hypoplasia and stippled epiphyses/malformed vertebral bodies.
- Other features include hydrocephalus, microcephaly, IUGR, eye abnormalities and postnatal developmental delay.

## M2.10 Answers

**A** True.
**B** True.
**C** True.
**D** True.

Note:
- High risk of mortality (>25%) is associated with pulmonary hypertension, coarctation of the aorta – complicated, Marfan's syndrome with aortic involvement, hypertrophic obstructive cardiomyopathy.

## M2.11 Answers

**A** True.
**B** True.
**C** True.
**D** True.

Note: Complications of septic miscarriage:
- Crepitus may occur following infection with gas-forming organisms – this usually complicates illegal abortions.
- Endometritis progressing to pelvic cellulitis/abscess and septicaemia.
- Endotoxic shock – features include hypotension, tachycardia, tachypnoea, hypothermia (<35°C) or pyrexia, hypoxaemia, oliguria and positive blood cultures.

## M2.12 Answers

**A** True.
**B** True.
**C** False – Not associated with paternal age.
**D** False – MSAFP low.

Note:
- 55% of neonates with Down syndrome have structural anomaly – cardiac anomalies (atrioventricular canal defects), GI (duodenal atresia, exomphalos, Hirschprung's disease), urinary tract/limb defects (fifth finger clinodactily), congenital cataract.

## M2.13 Answers

**A** True.
**B** False.
**C** False.
**D** False.

Note:

- Causes of raised MSAFP: wrong dates (underestimation), multiple pregnancy, abdominal wall defects, upper GI obstruction, congenital nephrosis, placental/cord tumours, obstructive uropathy, feto-maternal haemorrhage, CAML, sacro-coccyteal terratoma, maternal liver disease, smoking, Afro-Caribbean ethnic background.

## M2.14 Answers

**A** **True** – Associated with increased risk of diabetes mellitus, osteoporosis, scoliosis and emphysema.
**B** **False** – Infertility is universal except in mosaics. Not improved by testosterone.
**C** **False** – Not associated with impaired sense of smell (Kallman's syndrome).
**D** **False** – Features include poorly developed secondary sexual characteristics, small testicles, gynaecomastia, increased height.

## M2.15 Answers

**A** **True** – Associated with increased nuchal transluscency, coarctation of the aorta, atrial septal defects, cystic hygroma, fetal hydrops.
**B** **True** – Increased risk of systemic hypertension.
**C** **True** – Increased risk of Hashimoto's thyroiditis.
**D** **False** – There is *hypo*plasia of the nails and short fourth metacarpals.

## M2.16 Answers

**A** False.
**B** True.
**C** **True** – Associated with posterior urethral valves in males and urgent assessment required in males with an enlarged bladder.
**D** True.

Note:

- Pelvicalyceal dilatation identifies fetuses requiring postnatal urological assessment (renal scan at about 1 week of age) + prophylactic antibiotics as risk of vesicoureteric reflux.

## M2.17 Answers

**A** **False** – Clitoral enlargement is a sign of virilization and does not occur in PCOS.
**B** **True** – Menstrual abnormalities – amenorrhoea/oligomenorrhoea/irregular bleeding.
**C** **True.**
**D** **True.**

## M2.18 Answers

**A** **True.**
**B** **True.**
**C** **True.**
**D** **False.**

Note:
- Phenytoin, cortisone, minoxidil, diazoxide, cyclosporin A alter the texture and extent of hair growth – the pattern is non-androgenic and is referred to as hypertrichosis.

## M2.19 Answers

**A** **True** – 10% have hyperprolactinaemia.
**B** **False.**
**C** **True** – 25% have hyperprolactinaemia.
**D** **True** – Associated with increased TRH, which stimulates prolactin release.

Note:
- Hyperprolactinaemia is associated with: prolactin-secreting adenomas, lactotroph hyperplasia, acromegaly, Cushing's disease, empty sella syndrome, primary hypothyroidism.

## M2.20 Answers

**A** **False** – FSH and LH levels are low and may be undetectable.
**B** **True** – Pituitary response to GnRH is suboptimal but regained at ~15% below the ideal body weight and occurs before the resumption of menses.
**C** **True.**
**D** **False** – Prolactin is normal.

## M2.21 Answers

**A** **True.**
**B** **True.**
**C** **True.**
**D** **False** – Kallman's syndrome causes *primary* amenorrhoea.

## M2.22 Answers

**A** False.
**B** False.
**C** True.
**D** True.

Note:

- Stage I – Limited to the ovaries: Ia – one ovary, capsule intact, no ascites; Ib – both ovaries, capsules intact, no ascites; Ic – capsule breached or ascites.
- Stage II – Presence of peritoneal deposits in pelvis: IIa – On uterus or tubes.
- Stage IV – Distant metastases including intrahepatic.

## M2.23 Answers

**A** **False** – Carboplatin causes less nausea and vomiting, renal or ototoxicity than cisplatin.
**B** **True** – Platinum agents are direct renal tubular toxins. Renal damage is the major dose-limiting toxicity and is associated with hypomagnesaemia. Renal damage can be reduced by forced diuresis using saline or mannitol or by administration in hypertonic saline.
**C** **True** – Nausea and vomiting can be reduced by use of 5-HT antagonist ondansetron, H2 antagonists and corticosteroids.
**D** **True.**

## M2.24 Answers

**A** **False** – Endometrial cancer should be managed surgically by TAH + BSO because of the risk of adnexal involvement.
**B** **False** – The evidence is that excision of vaginal cuff does not reduce the risk of vault recurrence.
**C** **False** – The value and risks of HRT remain controversial.
**D** **False** – There is no evidence that tubal ligation or insertion of a cervical suture reduced the risk of pelvic or vault recurrence.

## M2.25 Answers

**A** **False** – Depth of invasion is the most important prognostic indicator.
**B** **True.**
**C** **False** – Prognosis is similar to melanomas elsewhere.
**D** **False** – Manage surgically. Radiotherapy is ineffective and adjuvant chemotherapy and immunotherapy have no proven value.

**M2.26 Answers**

    **A** **True.**

    **B** **True** – Chemosensitive with 82% cured. Results of radical surgery are poor.

    **C** **False** – Clear cell adenocarcinoma of the vagina is related to in utero exposure to DES.

    **D** **True** – Present with vaginal bleeding and a grape-like mass in the vagina.

**M2.27 Answers**

    **A** **False** – Failure rate (Pearl index – failure rate per 100 woman-years) = 0.1 if correctly taken.

    **B** **True** – COPC use is associated with an increase in the risk of developing breast cancer (relative risk 1.24 in current users).

    **C** **False** – In women who smoke, COCP should be stopped at the age of 35 years.

    **D** **True** – Valproate does not induce hepatic enzymes.

**M2.28 Answers**

    **A** **True** – If strings are visible, device should be removed – 50% reduction in spontaneous miscarriage rate.

    **B** **False** – Not teratogenic.

    **C** **True.**

    **D** **True** – Risk of third stage complications such as PPH is increased.

Note:

* Increased risk of ectopic pregnancy 1:25.

**M2.29 Answers**

    **A** **True** – Mifepristone is a glucocorticoid antagonist. It inhibits negative feedback of cortisol on ACTH secretion resulting in a significant increase in ACTH and cortisol after single 100 mg dose.

    **B** **False.**

    **C** **True** – Acts on the high concentration of progesterone receptors in decidua resulting in withdrawal of progesterone support.

    **D** **True** – Increases uterine concentrations of prostaglandins (probably by inhibiting prostaglandin metabolism) and also increases the sensitivity of the myometrium to prostaglandins.

**M2.30 Answers**

    **A** **True** – $MgSO_4$ is superior to diazepam or phenytoin in the treatment of eclampsia.

    **B** **False** – The loading dose of $MgSO_4$ should be administered over 5–10 minutes.

    **C** **False** – Recurrent seizures should be treated with a bolus dose of 2 g.

    **D** **True.**

### M2.31 Answers

**A** **False** – Planned C/S is not associated with significant increase in maternal morbidity compared to planned vaginal delivery.
**B** **True.**
**C** **False** – Lovset's manoeuvre is used for delivery of upper limbs.
**D** **False** – After-coming head is delivered manually or with Neville–Barnes forceps.

### M2.32 Answers

**A** **True** – Elective defibulation around 20 weeks' gestation reduces lacerations and avoids lacerations and anterior episiotomy in labour.
**B** **False** – If re-infibulation after delivery is requested, it should be made clear that the procedure is illegal in the UK. The consequences of more scarring and subsequent sexual and reproductive difficulties should be explained.
**C** **True** – Obstetric complications include wound infection and retention of lochia causing puerperal sepsis.
**D** **False** – During delivery, an anterior or midline episiotomy should be performed.

### M2.33 Answers

**A** **True.**
**B** **True.**
**C** **False.**
**D** **True.**

Note: Indications for echocardiography:
- Family history of cardiac anomaly.
- Increased nuchal translucency.
- Maternal disease – IDDM/PKU/connective tissue disease.
- Exposure to teratogens – phenytoin/isotrentinoin/lithium.
- Fetal infection – rubella/parvovirus/coxsackie.
- Prior identification of other fetal anomaly.

### M2.34 Answers

**A** **True** – Treatment with metronidazole has been shown to improve outcome only in women with bacterial vaginosis and a previous spontaneous preterm delivery.
**B** **True** – Bacterial products such as collagenase may weaken the fetal membranes, causing PPROM.
**C** **True** – Tocolytics should not be used in the presence of evidence of intrauterine infection and are less likely to be effective.
**D** **True** – Erythromycin crosses the placenta readily and is ideal for antenatal antibiotic prophylaxis.

## M2.35 Answers

**A** True.

**B** False – Hyperglycaemia in diabetics.

**C** True – CVS side effects include maternal and fetal tachycardia, hypotension, palpitations, arrhythmias, chest pain, pulmonary oedema.

**D** True.

## M2.36 Answers

**A** True – Malignant or pre-malignant endometrial conditions should be excluded and the uterus should be <12 weeks' size.

**B** False – Failed response to IUS is not a contraindication.

**C** True – Pre-operative counselling and patient selection is vital – women should not expect amenorrhoea.

**D** True – The effect on dysmenorrhoea remains uncertain – some practitioners consider dysmenorrhoea as a contraindication to endometrial ablation/resection. Others suggest that 'true dysmenorrhoea' is significantly improved in most women.

## M2.37 Answers

**A** True – Treatment with GnRH agonists should be limited to 6 months as there is loss of 6% of bone mineral density after a 6-month course.

**B** False – Bone mineral density is restored 2 years after cessation of therapy.

**C** False – Combined oral contraceptives, progestogens, danazol and GnRH agonists are equally effective in relieving endometriosis-related pain but with different side effect profiles.

**D** False – GnRH agonists are inactive on oral administration.

## M2.38 Answers

**A** False – The majority (~80%) of DVTs in pregnancy occur in the left leg.

**B** False – Commoner in multiparous women.

**C** False – Blood group O is protective.

**D** False – In pregnancy, below-knee DVTs should be treated.

## M2.39 Answers

**A** False – Rheumatoid arthritis typically improves in pregnancy.

**B** False – Sarcoidosis is unaffected or may improve during pregnancy.

**C** False – Asthma may improve, worsen (typically severe disease) or remain unchanged.

**D** False – Eczema often, but not invariably, improves in pregnancy.

### M2.40 Answers

**A** **False** – Typically presents in the third trimester with malaise, anorexia, nausea and vomiting and epigastric pain and profound hypoglycaemia.
**B** **True** – More common in primigravidae.
**C** **False.**
**D** **True** – Obstetric cholestasis is associated with antepartum and intrapartum fetal distress.

Note:
• More common with male fetuses (3x).

### M2.41 Answers

**A** **False** – Associated with lower MSAFP, beta HCG and uE3.
**B** **True.**
**C** **True.**
**D** **True** – Preterm delivery is increased, both iatrogenic (IUGR, macrosomia, PET/impaired renal function) or spontaneous (20% risk, hydramnios).

Note:
• The risk of aneuploidy is not increased.

### M2.42 Answers

**A** **False** – Folate deficiency may occur in sickle cell disease because of increased erythropoiesis. However, sickle cell anaemia does not respond to folic acid.
**B** **False** – Microcytosis is typical.
**C** **False** – Low MCV.
**D** **True** – Exchange transfusion may be used, especially in a crisis or if the woman presents late in pregnancy.

### M2.43 Answers

**A** **False** – Increased thyroid binding globulin.
**B** **False** – Increased total T4 and total T3.
**C** **True** – Free T4, free T3 and TSH remain unchanged.
**D** **False** – TSH is suppressed in hyperthyroidism.

### M2.44 Answers

**A** **True** – An intrauterine gestation sac is usually visualized by transvaginal scanning at HCG >1500 IU/L and by transabdominal scanning at HCG >6000 IU/L.
**B** **False** – A pseudo-sac is identified in 10–20% of ectopic pregnancies.
**C** **True** – In a normal intrauterine pregnancy, FH is always detectable at CRL >6 mm.
**D** **True** – In a normal intrauterine pregnancy, FH is always detectable if gestation sac diameter >30 mm.

## M2.45 Answers

A **False** – Lowest risk in 25–29 age group.

B **True** – Older reports show a wide variation in incidence worldwide – high in Far East 1:85 (Indonesia), lower in West 1.5:1000 live births (UK). More recent reports indicate that this difference is much less obvious.

C **False** – Recurrence risk of molar pregnancy = 1:76; 1:6.5 after two previous molar pregnancies.

D **True** – Malignant potential higher with complete mole – 16% require chemotherapy compared to 0.5% after partial mole.

## M2.46 Answers

A **False** – Initial HCG <3000 IU/L.

B **False** – The presence of fetal cardiac activity is a contraindication to medical treatment.

C **True** – Ectopic mass <3.5 cm.

D **False** – Maternal compromise (tachycardia/hypotension) is a contraindication.

## M2.47 Answers

A **False** – Transplacental spread of bacteria causes fetal infection.

B **True** – In pregnancy, presents with flu-like illness (two-thirds of women), GI symptoms, fever – often misdiagnosed as UTI or influenza.

C **True.**

D **False** – Late-onset neonatal disease occurs in term neonates after uncomplicated pregnancy and typically presents with meningitis.

## M2.48 Answers

A **False** – Bacteriuria should be treated in the antenatal period.

B **False** – Benzyl penicillin is the antibiotic of choice.

C **False** – Women with antenatal GBS bacteriuria should be treated with intrapartum antibiotics. Further screening is unnecessary.

D **True** – Antenatal bacteriuria is a risk factor for preterm delivery.

## M2.49 Answers

A **True.**

B **False** – Screen neonate for HIV infection by PCR at birth, 3 and 6 weeks and 6 months and with an HIV antibody test at 18 months.

C **True.**

D **True.**

## M2.50 Answers

**A False** – The micturiction reflex is induced by stretching of the bladder with afferent impulses transmitted via the pelvic splanchnic nerves to S2,3,4 (parasympathetic). Efferent impulses leave the spinal cord at S2,3,4 via parasympathetic pre-ganglionic fibres through the pelvic splanchnic nerves and inferior hypogastric plexuses to the bladder where they synapse with post-ganglionic neurons.

**B True** – External urethral sphincter comprises urogenital diaphragm and periurethral muscle fibres – skeletal muscles, which are under voluntary control.

**C True** – Micturiction is a reflex action controlled by higher centres in the cerebral cortex in toilet-trained individuals.

**D True.**

## M2.51 Answers

**A True** – Associated with reduced bladder capacity at cystometry and the presence of petechial haemorrhages at cystoscopy, especially on re-fill.

**B False** – Urine is typically sterile.

**C True** – Painful, ulcerating pan-cystitis occurring more commonly in women and presenting with lower abdominal pain, perineal discomfort dysuria, frequency, urgency and dyspareunia. Florid ulceration of the bladder mucosa is uncommon.

**D False** – Involuntary detrusor contractions are consistent with DI or hyperreflexia.

## M2.52 Answers

**A True.**

**B True.**

**C True.**

**D True.**

Note: Effects of raloxifene in post-menopausal women:

- Bone metabolism – osteo-protective and associated with increased bone mineral density and a significant reduction in vertebral fractures in osteoporotic women. Non-significant reduction in non-vertebral fractures.
- Breasts – antioestrogenic effects with a significant reduction in the risk of developing breast cancer.
- Reproductive tract – antioestrogenic effects. There is some evidence that this may translate into a reduction in the risk of endometrial cancer.

## M2.53 Answers

**A True** – Oestrogenic in post-menopausal reproductive tract. There is stimulation of fibroid growth, induction/re-activation of endometriosis and adenomyosis.

**B False** – Adjuvant tamoxifen in women with breast cancer is associated with a 50% reduction in recurrence and a 25% reduction in mortality.

**C False.**

**D True** – The risk of venous thromboembolism is increased 4.7–5.7-fold.

## M2.54 Answers

    **A** **True** – Maximum permitted exposure (MPE) levels are set by regulation to minimize the risk of injury to patients and staff.

    **B** **False** – The $CO_2$ laser is ideal for vaporization and as it is readily absorbed by water, it is not ideal for hysteroscopic surgery.

    **C** **True** – The Nd:YAG laser produces light in the near infrared part of the spectrum (invisible) which can be transmitted by a fibreoptic system. Greater depth of tissue penetration compared to $CO_2$ laser.

    **D** **True** – The argon laser produces light in the blue and blue–green part of the spectrum (visible). Commonly used in ophthalmology.

## M2.55 Answers

    **A** **False** – In women undergoing major surgery for malignancy, low dose heparin (5000 U b.d.) is not superior to 'no treatment' in preventing VTE. Heparin 5000 U 2 h pre-op plus 5000 U 8 hourly reduces the risk of VTE without increasing the risk of life-threatening haemorrhage.

    **B** **False.**

    **C** **False** – Heparin has a short half-life and its effects are more easily reversed with protamine sulphate.

    **D** **False** – Calf compression on its own does not reduce VTE risk in women undergoing major surgery for malignant disease.

## M2.56 Answers

    **A** **True** – Remnants of the mesonephric system in the female include the epoophron, paroophron and Gartner's duct.

    **B** **True.**

    **C** **False** – The hydatid of Morgani is a remnant of the Müllerian duct which forms a small cystic structure at the distal end of the fallopian tube.

    **D** **True.**

## M2.57 Answers

    **A** **False** – Haematocolpos is secondary to imperforate vagina/low vaginal atresia.

    **B** **True** – Presents with primary amenorrhoea, cyclical lower abdominal pain ± urinary retention.

    **C** **True.**

    **D** **False.**

Note:

- Haematocolpos is a lower abdominal mass on examination with imperforate membrane at the introitus which may be blue in colour + mass in vagina on PR examination.

### M2.58 Answers

**A** **False** – Physical inspection of genitalia in insufficient for sexual assignment and karyotype is essential.

**B** **True.**

**C** **True** – U&E essential – salt losing syndrome characterized by low $Na^+/Cl^-$ and raised $K^+$.

**D** **False** – In Turner's syndrome there are normal female genitalia at birth.

T - #1085 - 101024 - C0 - 229/152/17 - PB - 9781853157264 - Gloss Lamination